Eileen!
Many thanks and be well,
Do Enjoy!

EAT YOURSELF SUPER ,

Dr Todd

www.eatyourselfsuper.com/blog

EAT YOURSELF SUPER

...ONE BITE AT A TIME

*A Superfoods Journey
for the Happy, Healthy,
and Hungry*

TODD J. PESEK, M.D.

NEW YORK

EAT YOURSELF SUPER
...ONE BITE AT A TIME

A Superfoods Journey for the Happy, Healthy, and Hungry

by TODD J. PESEK, M.D.

ISBN 978-1-61448-167-6 Paperback
ISBN 978-1-61448-168-3 eBook
Library of Congress Control Number: 2012930437

Published by:
MORGAN JAMES PUBLISHING
The Entrepreneurial Publisher
5 Penn Plaza, 23rd Floor
New York City, New York 10001
(212) 655-5470 Office
(516) 908-4496 Fax
www.MorganJamesPublishing.com

Cover Design by:
Rachel Lopez
rachel@r2cdesign.com

Interior Design by:
Bonnie Bushman
bonnie@caboodlegraphics.com

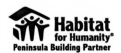

In an effort to support local communities, raise awareness and funds, Morgan James Publishing donates a percent of all book sales for the life of each book to Habitat for Humanity Peninsula and Greater Williamsburg.
Get involved today, visit
www.HelpHabitatForHumanity.org.

IMPORTANT NOTICE

The author and the publisher make no representation or warranties with respect to the accuracy or completeness of the contents of this work and specifically disclaim all warranties, including without limitation warranties of fitness for a particular purpose. No warranty may be created or extended by sales or promotional materials. The advice and strategies contained herein may not be suitable for every situation.

The information in this book is designed to provide health information for the purposes of reference and guidance and to accompany, not replace, the services of a qualified healthcare practitioner or physician. It is not the intent of the author or the publisher to recommend or prescribe any substance to cure, mitigate, treat, or prevent any disease. None of the statements in this book have been evaluated by the Food and Drug Administration. In the event you use this information with or without seeking medical attention, the author and publisher shall not be liable or otherwise responsible for any loss, damage, or injury caused or arising out of, directly or indirectly, by the information contained in this book or its use.

The recipes in this book are to be followed exactly as written. The author and/or publisher are not responsible for specific health or allergy concerns that may require medical supervision or for any adverse reactions to these recipes, foods or supplements.

While the author has made every effort to provide accurate telephone and Internet addresses at the time of publication, neither the author nor publisher assumes any responsibility for errors, or for changes that occur after publication.

DEDICATION

To my wife, Leah, and to my daughters, Kaia and Lily. You enrich and enlighten my journey in ways which cannot be communicated in words or anything short of infinite love.

To my elders, who selflessly give of their knowledge and wisdom.

To all my cosmic family. We are all brothers and sisters, every last being, we are all one. I honor the interconnectedness of us all.

To our children. All of our children, for it is from them who we have borrowed the land, sky, water and air. We must return these beings in all their beautiful, mystical majesty.

To you, for receiving this humble offering with an open heart.

CONTENTS

ACKNOWLEDGEMENTS

I wish to thank my many supporters, without whose help this work would not have been possible, from my family, friends, patients and colleagues to my many mentors and gurus the world over. You are too numerous to mention, but I know who you are and you know who you are. Additionally, I would like to thank my wife Leah J. Pesek for her support and assistance compiling our Superfoods kitchen recipes, and, my little sister, Sandra J. S Bean, for her invaluable assistance with manuscript preparation.

I am particularly indebted to the cosmos, earth and plants for their enrapturing majesty, and the shamans, bushmasters, healers, and elders, my guides through the aforementioned. You are the keepers of this treasure trove of knowledge, wisdom and enlightenment and continue, to this day, to keep me captivated with your age-old wisdom and warm smiles. I whole-heartedly express my love and gratitude to you all for so willingly and forthrightly giving your time and attention to teach me so that I may pass the knowledge as it coalesces with experience and manifests as wisdom in a multitude of applications. And, many, many thanks for the continued open door.

I will continue to do the same as promised.

INTRODUCTION
A Note from Dr. Todd

Hi, I'm Dr. Todd Pesek.

Let's start with a most important tenet: I love food! And you should, too. I am not here to tell you to have some sort of complicated relationship with your food. In fact, I am excited to share the news of how simple it is to be healthy! Your body knows what to do if you give it the right building blocks and fuel... just like a well-laid foundation provides stability to your home.

Where does my food-love come from? I spent the early part of my life as a rough-and-tumble little boy in the valleys and mountains of rural Appalachia. In this region, I grew to respect tradition and what, in reciprocal fashion, the Earth can do for all of us—heal and sustain, amuse and entertain, enlighten and nurture the spirit.

In tow with my elders, I learned my family's herbalist and root doctoring traditions, and on our self-sustaining farm, I learned to grow, harvest, gather and prepare real food! I learned the joy of a beautiful garden (my little sister and I were known to spend all day outside...snacking from the fields and forest for breakfast, lunch, and dinner!). I think back to the natural behaviors of kids set free outdoors and I realize that we know what we need to be healthy—sunshine, pure water, colorful foods, and being present and connected with nature as she inspires cosmic awe and illustrates lessons in resilience and the cycles of life. These are interspersed—of course—with lots of smiling, silliness and laughter. Life at its finest!

That little boy eventually grew up with these values in place. My elders and traditions lit within me a fire to learn from other elders and traditions in health and wellness from around the world. So, inspired by this passion and purpose, I took my first expeditionary trip to the jungles of Belize thirteen years ago. Since that time, I have worked and spoken in numerous countries, including Belize, India, Peru, Guatemala, Canada, the United States, and Ireland. I lived beside shamans and bushmasters in the jungle and other sacred places, and learned amid thousand-year-old healing spaces the world over. I have collaborated and studied with well-known medical doctors, scholars and researchers within some of the most prestigious hospitals in the United States.

Traditionally, I am an herbalist and root doctor. Academically, I am a medical doctor with an ethnobotanical scholarship focus—this means that I study plants and people. A natural outcropping of this is that I work to look at the relationships people have with plants and then I apply all of this as a holistic physician. Along the way, my journey has meant many different things from studying the plant compost of the ancient Maya civilization to see what they used as medicines hundreds of years ago, to studying with contemporary traditional healers the world over, to looking at how diet and foods affect my patients.

When eventually I settled down here and wound up faced with the decision of what I wanted to do in the medical field, the answer was obvious to me: I wanted to show people how to be well. I wanted to assist with a sustainable solution, not a quick-fix band-aid. This does not immediately reconcile with the current majority mindset in the Western medical community, but I knew that it was truth, and I wanted to help people to *truly* be in good health. I felt quite lucky to be able to do that by taking the experiences of my travels and ethnobotanical research, and combine all of this with my traditions and medical knowledge.

And so, after many years of extensive international research and practice experience in preventive, integrative, holistic health, I now specialize in disease prevention and reversal toward longevity and vital living—and I use food as a large part of that program.

As I moved from place to place, I saw many groups of people living strong, vital, healthy lives. They did not expect cancer or heart attacks. I wanted to know their secrets. They were usually not materially rich as a general rule. They did not drive fancy cars. They did not eat at fine restaurants three nights a week. But they were glowing with joy and strong with the life force all of us have as our birth-right. I was fortunate enough to study and learn their secrets, which aren't really secrets at all but rather a relatively simple set of practices.

Wellness and disease present themselves in every population, of all ages and in all areas of the planet. T. Colin Campbell, the researcher behind what is argu-ably the most comprehensive nutritional study of our time, The China Study, reflected on the diseases seen around the world. He coined them "Diseases of Affluence" and "Diseases of Poverty." These "Diseases of Affluence", or diseases of civilization, are the ones our Western society considers almost inevitable—heart disease, diabetes and cancer. These are seen in societies where there is relative wealth, because the diet followed then tends to change—and not for the better. But these are not a death sentence given to humans at birth. These are not guar-anteed. It does seem, however, that they are expected—and the treatments are oftentimes harmful and harsh.

Early in my medical career, I came upon a particular patient who was going to lose a portion of her bowel at the young age of eleven. I thought, this should not be happening. I stuck my neck out, and spoke up (a medical student in complete disagreement with the treatment plan). To make a long and complicated story short, through natural, dietary means, this surgery was avoided, and she is doing beautifully today. However, I was horrified that not only had this child gotten to this place (as many others have as well), but that modern medicine's best solution was to cut away the problem. The body can heal itself in remarkable ways if given the proper tools.

This is how I find myself now talking to you about the business of food. Be-cause Hippocrates' advice (for those who don't know, he was the father of modern medicine who lived some 2400 years ago), "let food by thy medicine and medi-cine by thy food" just so happens to hold completely true—our diets can provide us with not only the proper fuel to survive, but to thrive beautifully!

That may not seem like rocket science, but the Standard American Diet has quite a few people fooled into thinking they're getting what they need, when in fact, they're making themselves sick. It is essential that we understand this: the majority of cases of morbidity (in other words, diseases) simply need not exist. Not only are these diseases avoidable, but we can slow the progression or even reverse conditions already diagnosed.

It's fairly simple: our bodies are complex systems that best function in balance. When they are out of balance, disease results. The human body is equipped with the ability to change, adapt, equilibrate, and eliminate dangers to its systems. Your body CAN heal itself, when necessary...and I am beginning to see, increasingly, that it IS necessary for large numbers of tired, overweight, and otherwise suffering people.

The most common conditions are these diseases of civilization, which include arterial disease which leads to high blood pressure, heart attack and stroke; a broad range of autoimmune diseases; and inflammation, which plays a role in the aforementioned and leads to cancer and other pathologies. These are all manifestations of choices made on an ongoing basis—much of which involves our food.

I realize that this may be a shift in thinking. As a society, we tend to be reactionary rather than preventive, especially with regard to our bodies and medical care. We eat the fries as our vegetables and worry about the chest pains later on down the road. As that thought pattern begins to shift (and it IS shifting) to where it should be—equilibrium and prevention—we will begin to see a reduction in diseases of civilization and will live the lives of which we are capable: the Good Life.

To appreciate and strive toward the Good Life, we can learn from traditions that have sustained humanity for millennia. These traditions, which are alive in cultures throughout the world, offer us answers to complex questions of survivability, sustainability, holistic health and wellness, *joi de vivre*, and cultural and spiritual development—and in context of longevity and vital living.

So how can this book help you bring the knowledge of generations of healthy people the world over and the experience of a holistic medical doctor into your kitchen? Easy: with Superfoods.

In my clinical practice, I work to restore normal physiology for disease prevention and reversal, so my patients can live well and enjoy life to the fullest and most vital extent possible. I want the same for you! Superfoods are my preferred way to treat and reverse medical conditions in my office. You hold in your hands a toolbox to practice what I practice in my own life and the lives of those for whom I care. This book will help you begin your journey to wellness. I am excited to teach you how to Eat Yourself Super!

This book is intended to act as a guide for you on your journey as you wind your way around the perimeter of your grocery store, through the local farmer's market, into your Community Sponsored Agriculture box, or wherever it is you choose to procure the food you eat. Maybe even in the earth, shrubs, and trees that surround you!

So, read on. And here's my wish for you: <u>Eat Yourself Super—One Bite at a Time</u>.

Many thanks and be well,

Dr. Todd

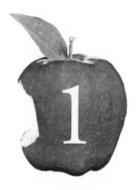

DISEASES OF CIVILIZATION: THE NOT INEVITABLE!

Since the beginning of our time on Earth, people have enhanced health by living in balance and in close connection with nature, engaging in physical and mental exercise and eating well. We have gotten further and further away from this lifestyle, and it is clearly harmful. A return to mindful living can pave the way to true wellness and vitality—and the understanding of global healing traditions can teach us a mindful way of life, including how and what to eat, and how we, as a society, can thrive in harmony with nature.

MISSED CONNECTIONS ON THE ROAD TO WELLNESS

A considerable part of what is missing from the Western Lifestyle is attention to how one negotiates the fine balance between modern human existence and our natural world. Especially in the current age, we are highly disconnected from nature, without which we would not survive. We spend inordinate amounts of time indoors, and as the electronic media empire expands, the problem grows. *There is no human health without environmental health* and this includes both social and natural worlds. It is up to us to create a harmonious situation in our environment in order to ensure continued good health.

As complex beings, we have a unique niche in our ecosystem that is all but ignored by extremely powerful forces around us: media and advertisements featuring the highest bidder, business and industry putting profit over human welfare, and educational institutions that promote skills over creativity and proffer junk food to our children (I am purposely leaving out modern healthcare, but I'll come back to that!).

It is about balance, which is not always the easy way, but always the most beneficial way of life. Without pure water, clean air, and nutritious food we cannot attain health. It is impossible to detoxify while taking in toxic-laden water, air, and food. It is impossible to be nutritionally complete from depleted soils. All of this is dependent upon the sustained health of our ecosystems and, ultimately, planet Earth.

We must work hard at restoring balance as the present generation—for the first time in recorded history of such—has a shorter life expectancy than the last. When comparing consumers in high-income countries like the United States, Japan, Sweden and France, those who eat the Standard American Diet (hereinafter referred to as the SAD) have lower life expectancies in general. Living the Superfoods lifestyle and helping our children to do so can help to ameliorate this catastrophic problem.

LEARNING FROM TRADITIONS

Back to the idea of global healing traditions. Because the natural world is the natural world anywhere it is, human cultures have common patterns. There are universal themes to health and healing the world over, and they are generally aligned with longtime practices—generations of health and wellness knowledge. In fact, approximately 80% of the world's population uses traditional health and wellness practices for their primary healthcare. These time-honored healing traditions have existed for millennia. I realize that there are those out there who think, "Traditional medicine? You mean I have to rub myself with leaves and eat an entire lemon the next time I get a cold?" This is a fallacious view. Traditional healing probably took place in your own mother's kitchen. Ever had herbal tea when you were under the weather? Honey for a sore throat? Crackers for an upset stomach?

All traditional remedies. But something most people don't realize is that much of modern medical practice is rooted in traditional healing practices as well. More than 25% of modern medications stem from traditional healing knowledge.

I'm not talking about some obscure medications used to treat rare conditions, but "blockbusters" used in front-line modern medicine the world over. Medications like aspirin, opioid painkillers, medications for high blood pressure and heart disease, cutting-edge medications for diabetes, some of the top anticancer medications, even medications and drugs that help make surgery possible—these all come from traditional healing knowledge and traditional knowledge of plants.

A Note from Dr. Todd:

Traditional medicine provides primary healthcare to roughly 80% of the worlds population. So, 80% never left traditional medicine. The other 20% of the world is now returning to traditional medicine in the form of Complementary and Alternative Medicine (CAM), which is rooted in traditions.

However, their current use is in contrast to the millennia of traditions which bore this knowledge in a complex shared learning experience with the natural world. Think of it this way: modern medicine is relatively new; it has only been around for a couple hundred years. As the new kid in town, the field seems to know no better than to isolate highly potent monocompounds from complex mixtures in plants and apply these to masking of symptoms without treating the underlying causes. There is little to no promotion of using the whole plant or to looking at the illness in a broader context. It is an isolated, reactionary system that is not sustainable.

Much more so than modern medicine, these traditional health and wellness practices honor the synergy within plants and nature; this system of heathcare spills over into the diet as well, because what we eat is intertwined with our health…and our ancestors knew it. It boggles my mind to see a physician writing prescriptions for medications to treat symptoms which can be reversed with food right then (rather than developing into a life threatening condition) operating under the mask of very profitable pharmaceutical treatment. Interested business has played way too prominent a role in standard of care medicine and medical education—and that is a large part of the problem.

THE DISEASE EPIDEMIC

Our nation is in the midst of a catastrophic heath crisis of our own doing. By consuming the 20th century inaugurated SAD and losing touch with our roots, we are making ourselves sick. The major diseases of civilization include arterial disease (which, for our discussion, includes high blood pressure and atherosclerosis and leads to heart disease, heart attack, stroke, and other circulatory compromise), diabetes (the common type 2), and other pathologies rooted in inflammation; these plague our nation and indeed the world as other countries shift to the SAD. <u>The reality is, the majority of cases of these diseases need not exist.</u>[1-6] They can be prevented through changes to diet and lifestyle. Moreover, oftentimes, if these diseases do exist, they are actually reversible.[7-9]

A Note from Dr. Todd:

Know this: The majority of cases of morbidity, or disease, simply need not exist!

Specifically, arterial disease—which leads to heart disease, heart attack and stroke—is resultant from an overconsumption of fats or lipids. Arterial disease drives, but is also caused by, inflammation. Diabetes (type 2) is resultant from an overconsumption of sugars, but it is also exacerbated by an over consumption of fat—these both feed into inflammation. Maladies brought on by chronic inflammation include cancer, the gamut of autoimmune diseases and even other ailments such as certain neurological diseases like Multiple Sclerosis and Alzheimer's. The science is clear, the mountains of data have spoken, and research irrefutably demonstrates that occurrences of diseases of civilization are preventable or even reversible by simply avoiding what drives them and working to combat chronic inflammation by shifting from the SAD to a healthful diet.

Let's start at the beginning. Our ancestors evolved with necessary fat and sugar cravings—these things are in relatively short supply in nature, and contain essential properties for energy and optimal health. However, at that time, they existed only in forms that are useful and physiologically friendly to the body—for example; fats found easily in nature, say as tree nuts, are more often than not healthful fats in good proportions; they are rich in essential fatty acids all necessary for brain and organ development and to balance out the inflammatory response of the body to keep human health in check. Likewise, sugars in fruits are presented in a nice little package with fiber and other phytonutrients, so the sugar is not absorbed into the blood stream too quickly and thus result in a blood sugar elevation.

Note from Dr. Todd:

Fruit has fructose, which has been vilified due to the highly processed, health mortifying high fructose corn syrup (HFCS). Contrary to this highly processed distant relative, the concentrations of fructose in fruit are quite healthful for reasons mentioned above. High concentrations of fructose as in HFCS are horrible for you because fructose bypasses a key regulatory checkpoint in sugar metabolism. Basically, it gets processed even if processing is not needed, or even detrimental.

So, our ancestors craved these items, and when they were able to find them, they'd eat them. Fat and sugar contributed to the overall energy levels and wellness of the individual. Craving these items kept early woman and man energized and well.

Fast forward to now. We have ready access to highly refined fats and sugars, and we can't shut down that drive to consume them. Hence, these compounds are addictive—so they are consumed on levels of toxicity. The amounts consumed by modern woman and man are poisonous to us. Arterial disease manifests from eating too much fat—fat that our body cannot use. Diabetes results from eating too much sugar—sugar that our body cannot use. And, it all drives inflammation!

I witness it as I walk around in my daily life, and I'd bet that you do as well—overweight, tired, sick people are everywhere we go. Many, many individuals live with chronic conditions, diminishing the overall quality of life and wasting billions of dollars each year in the name of managing these conditions in our troubled healthcare system. It's a shame that many are not exploring the options for health that real foods can offer them. In a multitude of studies conducted over the past 10 years, Dean Ornish, M.D., has demonstrated that people with severe heart disease were able to halt progression and reverse it without drugs or surgery by making comprehensive lifestyle and dietary changes. These changes include stress management through meditation and yoga, smoking cessation, moderate exercise, good social support, and—tada!—dietary changes in the form of a low-fat, plant-based diet. These trials were published in major medical journals including the Journal of the American Medical Association.[4,8] Caldwell Esselstyn,

Jr., M.D., has further shown that one can arrest and reverse even severe heart disease with a ZERO fat, plant-based dietary intervention alone![2,3,7]

I have the benefit of the experience of breaking (real) bread with and studying multiple cultures with significant longevity; these cultures tend towards the diets of their ancestors. As Western culture became "civilized" in the last century or so, we have gotten further and further away from leaning this way ourselves. This was a huge mistake. There is nothing civilized about food that is so highly processed, there is no "food" left in it. This is exactly what is happening on our grocery store shelves and what is being served in countless homes.

INFLAMMATION

Chronic inflammation precipitates disease (Figure 1). Inflammation does have an important role in bodily function; it helps us recover from injury and fights off illness. However, in health, there must be balance between inflammation and anti-inflammation. The problems occur when there is chronic inflammation (scale leaning toward inflammation—a lack of balance) where it is not necessary for function. What we eat results in chronic inflammation in the body.

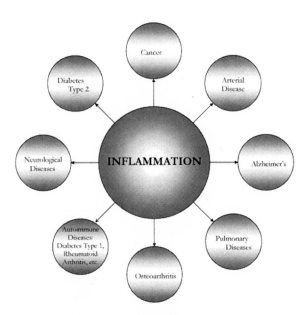

Figure 1. Inflammation, a vital physiologic function, drives the diseases of civilization when the scales are tipped toward chronic inflammation.

This is a well-known reality and sadly, this is not new news. In fact, the cover of *Time* Magazine's February 23, 2004 issue screamed, <u>The Secret Killer: The surprising link between inflammation and heart attacks, cancer, Alzheimer's and other diseases.</u>[6] We have known about the inflammation link for over a decade, and although pharmaceutical companies may be looking at developing more medications to throw at this problem, this won't provide the harmonious benefits that something else, something healthier, cheaper, and simpler, will. Plainly put, there is a better way. Superfoods can reduce or eliminate chronic inflammation and other illness-promoting conditions.

ARTERIAL DISEASE

We take in so much fat, the body says, "Wait! What do I do with all of this?" For clarity, by *fat*, I am referring to lipids which include triglycerides, phospholipids and cholesterol, for the most part. The term fat actually refers to neutral fat, which is another way of saying triglyceride, but "fat" has infiltrated mainstream media and in general has come to mean lipids. Also, I will mention here that, in my view, cholesterol has been unnecessarily blacklisted. We need it for health. Cholesterol is synthesized endogenously in our cells and is necessary for a number of important functions including cell membrane fluidity, digestion and the production of hormones. Cholesterol is actually the "father" of all hormones including testosterone, estrogen and vitamin D. The problem seems to arise with boatloads of exogenous cholesterol along with all the other lipids or fat which is taken in through diet into an imbalanced and toxic system. For the vast history of humanity, the majority of cholesterol came from endogenous synthesis. Add to the above, modern human's dietary load of sugar and other no-no's in context of systemic imbalance and it becomes too much…you get the picture.

Excessive exogenous dietary fat is eventually deposited into the vascular intimae (basically under the vascular lining), which, to make a long process short, causes atherosclerosis (the formation of fat laden plaques in the vessels) and inflammation

A Note from Dr. Todd:

Arterial disease—and all it brings —is fat toxicity.

and occludes healthful blood flow (Figure 2). Over time, due to plaque build up, inflammation, and endothelial (delicate innermost layer of cells in vessels) dysfunction there develops an inability of the vessels to repair, constrict, dilate—and carry out other functions necessary for health. Ultimately, this results in restriction to blood flow and, in essence, a clogging of the artery. This state (Figure 3) leads to life-threatening conditions including heart disease and heart attack, stroke, circulation disorders, high blood pressure, clotting and aneurism. Superfoods offer hope for those who suffer from arterial disease.

Normal Artery

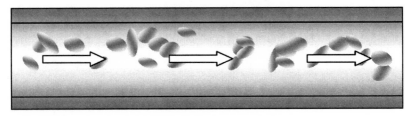

Normal blood flow

Atherosclerosis Artery

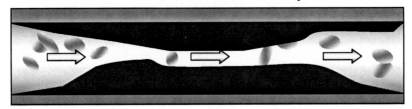

Plaque narrows artery, creating obstacle to normal blood flow

Figure 2. The process of atherosclerosis or deposition of fat in the vascular lining causes a restriction to blood flow, and drives inflammation. This is fat toxicity.

Stages of Atherosclerosis

Healthy Artery

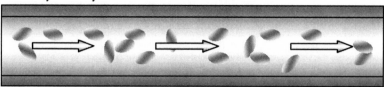

Build up begins

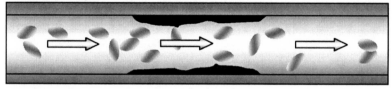

Plaque forms

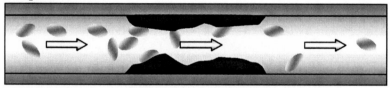

Plaque ruptures, blood clot forms

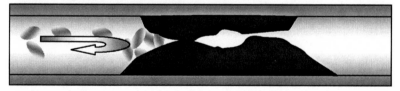

Figure 3. Over time, the process of atherosclerosis slowly diminishes blood flow and atherosclerotic plaques can rupture and have a blood clot form on them and thus completely occlude blood flow—if this occurs in the vasculature of the heart it is a heart attack, if in the brain a certain type of stroke.

The body is an amazing entity, in that it has all sorts of mechanisms for naturally repairing, rejuvenating, and detoxifying itself to effect healing. This involves a variety of processes, but, in this context, one such process stands out. It involves something called Endothelial Progenitor Cells (EPC). These cells have the ability to fix the vascular lining in the human body. At first, their very existence was hotly refuted, but they are now a commonplace topic in cardiac research.

What has been found through a variety of research studies is that these cells can facilitate repair of diseased arterial tissue—and that we can increase the amount of these cells at work in the body with Superfoods. In one such study, <u>Dietary intervention with Okinawan vegetables increased circulating endothelial progenitor cells in healthy young women</u>[10], participants simply ate more vegetables over a two week period, and showed marked increases of these cells in the body, as well as other healthful benefits. Interestingly, in studies on EPC, the high-fat, high-protein, low-carb fad diets are shown to be quite deleterious to the health, as these diets are high-fat, so they accelerate atherosclerosis, AND they potentially reduce the number of endothelial progenitor cells active in the body.[11]

A Note from Dr. Todd:

Your elders were right.
Eat your veggies!

DIABETES

There are two types of diabetes: type 1 and type 2. They have to do with sugar balance and sugar handling, in particular glucose, in our bodies. Tantamount to this sugar balance and handling are the amounts of sugar we consume, and the amount and function of insulin in our bodies. Insulin response is the key. Insulin is an essential protein necessary for glucose transport from the blood (where it goes from our food) into our cells (where it must go to be utilized for its primary function—production of energy, or cellular fuel for us to be active). If it hangs out in the blood too long it causes problems through glycation.

Type 1 diabetes results from an autoimmune attack on pancreatic islet cells which produce insulin. The net effect of this attack is less insulin function due to lower amounts of insulin in the body. This is an autoimmune process and, like all inflammatory conditions, could-well be reversible. I do have direct clinical experience reversing type 1 diabetes through holistic treatment such as the principles illustrated in this book. However, type 2 is the type generally induced by excessive sugar consumption and so when I speak of diabetes reversal, I am for the most part referring to type 2.

Type 2 is the most common type of diabetes. Per the American Diabetes Association,

> "In type 2 diabetes, either the body does not produce enough insulin or the cells ignore the insulin. Insulin is necessary for the body to be able to use glucose for energy. When you eat food, the

body breaks down all of the sugars and starches into glucose, which is the basic fuel for the cells in the body. Insulin takes the sugar from the blood into the cells. When glucose builds up in the blood instead of going into cells (they react and attach themselves to places they shouldn't [i.e., glycation]), this leads to diabetes complications." [12,13]

In essence, the body does not produce enough insulin (despite trying to do so) to shunt the toxic amounts of sugar we consume into our cells. Further, our cells get sick and tired of the insulin telling them to take in more sugar when they cannot—so they ignore even larger than normal levels of insulin and leave the sugar in the blood. The excessive fat throws things off too. The net effect of this elevated blood sugar is more glycation products and the deleterious health effects they cause (Figure 4).

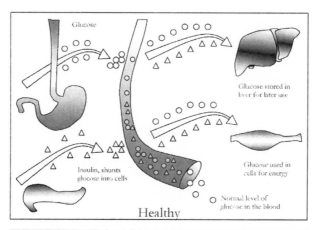

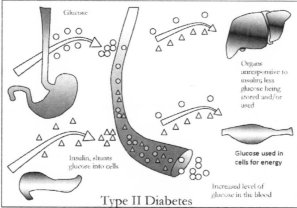

Figure 4. Diabetes or Sugar Toxicity

So you see, just as the fats get deposited in the vascular intimae, which drives disease, so too does something similar happen with the consumption of toxic levels of sugar. The body doesn't know what to do with these large amounts of excess sugar and biochemistry takes over. These sugars begin attaching to proteins and cellular proteins in blood in a non-mediated, basically haphazard process. An overwhelming body of evidence continues to suggest that glycation is an important pathogenic mediator of almost all diabetes complications. For example, glycation products are found in retinal (or eye) vessels of people with diabetes, and the levels of which correlate to levels of available glucose, glycation products in blood, and importantly with the severity of eye disease.[13]

A Note from Dr. Todd:

Diabetes is sugar toxicity.

Notably, one of the hallmarks in diabetes diagnostic criteria is a glycated hemoglobin (HgBA1c) which gives a running average of blood sugar levels based on the amount of sugars hanging on one's hemoglobin proteins in blood. Another test is "insulin resistance", assessed by elevated insulin levels. This occurs in diabetes type 2 because the body produces more insulin to deal with an overabundance of sugar (insulin levels can be detected with a lab test); this physiologic protective mechanism is eventually overcome though as the insulin levels cannot continue to go up but the sugar consumption and addiction can. Basically, the pancreas gives up. Let's reflect for a moment to realize the gravity of this situation. Glucose is our body's main source for short-term energy, but current evidence demonstrates that it is also responsible for the fueling of long-term diabetes complications. These complications occur mainly in the form of oxidants and pro-inflammatory glycation products.[13] It is a conundrum; a double-edged sword—we need sugar for fuel, so we crave it. It is

A Note from Dr. Todd:

Foods which are commonly consumed after being exposed to heat, i.e., cooked foods, contain a more significant amount of preformed glycation products—a crucial fact that offers a new perspective on cooked food as a major environmental risk factor.[13] In other words, we need to eat more raw greens, veggies, fruits, nuts and seeds for optimal health. Raw Superfoods are the cornerstone of a healthful diet.

more available, so we are eating more and do less physical activity to utilize it. Simple solution: eat less and be more active.

CANCER

Cancers are of all different etiologies, but the basis is the same as the other afore-mentioned diseases of civilization—inflammation. As we have discussed, inflammation is driven by the foods that we eat and the toxicities to which we are exposed in other ways. We can significantly lower the number of cancer diagnoses in the Western world by eating to reduce inflammation and eliminate toxins— Superfoods do just that.

While a full consideration of toxins and environmental interrelations in cancer, inflammation and health are outside the scope of this book, it is useful for us mention a few key realities here both as they relate to food specifically and indirectly.

A growing body of evidence demonstrates a multitude of established and suspected environmental exposures are in fact linked to genetic, reproductive, immune, endocrine and even behavioral dysfunctions which can ultimately lead to cancer and other adverse health effects.[14,15,16] In fact, it is estimated that 25%-33% of the global disease burden can be linked to environmental factors.[14,17,18]

In 2004, Environmental Working Group conducted a study in collaboration with Commonweal, an environmental research organization, where two major laboratories documented an average of 200 industrial toxicants in umbilical cord blood from 10 babies who were born August to September 2004 in United States hospitals. These tests demonstrated the presence of 287 chemicals, 180 of which cause cancer, 217 of which are neurotoxic, and 208 of which cause birth defects and developmental abnormalities. What is even more disturbing though is the fact that the combined effects of these toxins have not been studied.[19]

The Experimental Man Project is another good example which illustrates our ongoing environmental debacle. This project is a scientific study on the presence and effect of toxins upon the genes and the physiology of one man who has elected to undergo extensive testing. Thus far, out of 320 toxins for which he has been tested, 165 have come back with positive results.[20] From these extensive research efforts science is once again strongly corroborating common sense—toxins are toxic (going out on a limb there, right?) and, therefore, bad for us.

A few more which may surprise you:

- Mercury, which is a toxic heavy metal that has been banned from thermometers and the environment, continues to be put in peoples' mouths in the form of dental amalgams (if you have these you should consider having them removed by a qualified biological dentist—make sure they take necessary precautions to prevent further exposures during removal). This is an interesting one. Another is cadmium which is an extremely toxic heavy metal known to cause cancer, yet it is used in many consumer goods including batteries, paints, even jewelry for children.

- Toxic water? City water contains chlorine and its byproducts added as a disinfectant, plus a number of other chemicals, heavy metals, and other toxins which find their way in there due to runoff from pesticides, herbicides, and even refrigerants. These compounds have been linked to a multitude of pathologies including breast cancer.[21] Fluoride, which is added to drinking water in the United States, is another toxin of epic proportions—a caustic neurotoxin and endocrine disruptor, added to our drinking water!

- Toxic food, too?? In 2005, the FDA reported finding chlorinated pesticides in 63% of foods surveyed. Pesticides, herbicides and fungicides in food, often petrochemicals, have been linked to many types of cancers.[21]

- Yes, even the air. United States industrial facilities released 4.7 billion pounds of toxins into the air in 2005—72 million pounds of which are known carcinogens. Among the egregious atrocities are coal-fired power plants which spew nitrates, sulphates, and mercury into the air. These toxins have indeed been linked to greater than twenty thousand premature deaths annually.[21]

The Superfoods diet and lifestyle is anti-cancer because it not only reduces exposure to toxic substances, but it also helps eliminate predisposition to cancer by relieving the body of some of the toxic load which could put us all at risk for this diagnosis.

While you do not exist in a toxic free world at present, with some effort, YOU can approach as toxic free a state as possible. You must avoid as many toxins as you

reasonably can and you must undergo regular
cleansing periodically, just as your ancestors
have done before you (only sometimes for different reasons, such as abundance and famine!).

A Note from Dr. Todd:

Work toward a toxin free you!

Superfoods are the beginning of the journey in this regard as Superfoods, when
done right, are sustenance without toxicity—they are actually detoxifying even as
we will see!

THYROID

I realize fully that a comprehensive discourse on the endocrine system and hormonal function is not pertinent here, as is even a comprehensive picture of the
thyroid gland for that matter. However, it is useful for us to consider some extremely relevant points.

As you know, the body functions as a complex physiologic system in balance
(it is, however, an open system as it continuously interacts with its environment).
Much of this balance, or homeostasis, is affected by hormones—your endocrine
system. It functions in concert with your nervous system; this drives your physiologic symphony and keeps your internal environment constant in the face of
constantly changing external environmental parameters. When internal imbalance occurs, manifestations of this imbalance build up over time and eventually
this imbalance becomes known as disease.

I am sure you have heard hyperthyroid this, or hypothyroid that and probably know that there are a multitude of names for a bewilderingly complex array
of categorizations given to thyroids that are out of whack and under-functioning
(as in hypothyroidism), or over functioning (as in hyperthyroidism). It is more
common that the gland under-functions but the over-functioning gland is fairly
common as well. In a nutshell, this is a consequence of, you guessed it: toxicity
and our environment. I do have direct clinical experience reversing both under
and over functioning thyroid glands through holistic treatment based on Superfoods and the principles outlined in this book. It can be done!

Your thyroid's role is to tell every cell in your body how quickly to utilize or
metabolize sugar in producing energy for itself and the organism at large—you. It
is the knob that turns your metabolism up or down. It does so via secreting thyroid hormones in response to thyroid stimulating hormone which is secreted by

the pituitary gland in the brain. As we utilize sugar, we do so a bit inefficiently—with just about 40% of the energy stored in the chemical bonds of the sugar being captured and used as the sugar is metabolized. The remaining energy is dissipated toward our environment in the form of heat—this loss of heat is recorded as our basal body temperature and registers at about 98.6 degrees Fahrenheit.

If our metabolism is cranked up, as in the case of our immune system needing more energy to fight off an infection for example, we become febrile. Fever is a side effect of the increased metabolism precipitated by the need for increased energy to fight the infection. This is governed by the thyroid gland through its hormones which are comprised of various combinations of iodinated tyrosine (iodine atoms attached to an amino acid). In hypothyroid, or slow/under-functioning thyroid, things slow down, including energy levels. A patient with this condition presents with fatigue, goiter (swelling thyroid, which resides at base of neck) increased sensitivity to cold (cold hands and feet), constipation, brittle hair and nails (not growing, but breaking), dry skin, and difficulty losing weight. In hyperthyroid, or fast/over functioning thyroid, things speed up, including energy levels. Patients present with insomnia, goiter, heart palpitations/rapid heart beat, increased sensitivity to heat, sweating, diarrhea, and weight loss. This is a dangerous state because of the heart rhythm and rate possibilities.

So we've just thrown another edge onto this sugar sword—we need sugar for fuel, but many are eating more than their need on top of doing less physical activity to utilize all this sugar. Now, if you throw thyroid issues into the mix, many are metabolically underactive and therefore unable to utilize the sugar even if they needed it. Further, the fats get deposited faster as well—this accelerates arterial disease. What to do? Eat less, do more, and support the thyroid with Superfoods!

The thyroid needs a number of nutrients for optimal function. Two of the most important are iodine (which is an essential element in the halogen group), and tyrosine, which is an amino acid. These two are the building blocks of thyroid hormones. Another crucially important element is selenium—suffice it to say, for now, that we get these essentials in our food. Iodine is of particular importance to us given the fact that our ancestors got a lot more iodine in their diets than contemporary man and woman. Iodine deficiency is generally accepted as one of the top causes of preventable brain damage worldwide.

Iodine concentrates in soil and water. You get it from food grown in healthy, non-depleted soil and water ecosystems. It is particularly abundant in various greens, legumes, and root veggies and it is extremely concentrated in seaweed—of which our ancestors ate plenty. Not only is there less iodine in modern diets, but there are other halogens that look like iodine, but don't function like iodine, saturating our environments and therefore, our bodies. The aforementioned additives in tap water, in particular chlorine and fluoride, as well as bromine, a preservative used commonly in baked goods, are good examples and all likely add to the problem of endocrine disruption. By ensuring adequate daily intake of iodine through Superfoods, we can ensure thyroid support.

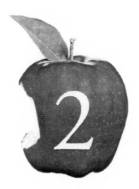

SECRETS OF LONG LIFE: A RETURN TO OUR ROOTS IN HEALTH

In essence, disease occurs via two routes: trauma and toxicity. Trauma is often a side effect of stress and a stressful pace of life—in a nutshell, a lack of present consciousness—rushing here, rushing there—I am sure you get the point. Be present and mindful. Also, do understand that we are profoundly traumatized by disconnection from the natural world—weather you realize it or not. Toxicity occurs in two varieties: physical toxins (in food and in environment) and mental toxins.

On toxic foods, a diet which is followed by two thirds of the world's population offers hope.[1] You can <u>Eat Yourself Super</u> through a diet which echoes that of your ancestors and those in a number of cultures worldwide who experience dramatically fewer cases of these diseases of civilization discussed earlier. Truly: change your diet and change your life. Eat foods which minimize toxicities (processed foods, herbicides, pesticides etc.) and avoid foods consumed on toxic levels, i.e., too much fat and sugar.

EPIGENETICS: GENES ARE NOT EQUAL TO PROMISES

On toxic thoughts, first things first: forget about your genes. They don't control you, you control them! They are controlled by your interaction with and perceptions of your environment—your beliefs.[22] it is no longer genetics, but rather epigenetics: how our environmental interactions, perceptions and beliefs control our genes and not vice versa.

Literally, our genes are a set of instructions completely incapable of turning themselves on or off; what turns them on or off are *you*, through perceptions and beliefs, and your environment. For the greater than 95% of the global human population who has a good set of genes, disease

> **A Note from Dr. Todd:**
>
> Your genes do NOT control you. You control them!

should not exist. It generally will not exist in the context of eliminated toxicities. Here is an interesting way to look at it: the well known, scientifically validated "placebo" and "nocebo" effects.

In placebo, positive thinking or belief that something will make you well, will make you well. In nocebo, negative thinking or belief that something will make you unwell, will make you unwell. Medical diagnoses given in and of themselves are oftentimes defeatist and the prospects of such impose a fear-based reality. I am strongly opposed to the use of medical diagnoses as an endpoint classification. Rather, if given, they should be given as a beginning point from where to work to improve (as best as one can). In my view, giving a diagnosis of diabetes type 2 or saying you are a "diabetic" or "you have diabetes" plants a self limiting construct which can become insurmountable—especially when coming from one's trusted physician. I would rather state it as:

> "Your body is breaking down under a toxic load of sugar. Therefore, you need to drastically cut or eliminate your consumption of sugar and foods which elevate your blood sugar, and eat more Superfoods. If you do not do so, you will begin to experience the complications of glycation which will insidiously rob you of your longevity and vitality—a condition referred to as diabetes."

You must manifest your intention of good health. To further illustrate this, of patients who have been given diagnoses, those that believe they will beat whatever ails them do so much more often than those who accept defeat from the outset. A few clinical stories come to mind here:

- A middle-aged and vibrantly glowing woman came into my office with a diagnosis (by needle biopsy) of invasive ductal carcinoma of the right breast. She said that she was going to beat it and asked of my assistance. I saw it in her eyes, her spirit spoke volumes. I knew that she would beat it—and she did without ANY conventional medical treatments. She did not have surgery, chemotherapy or radiation. She beat it with Superfoods, and a few other alternative medicine strategies.

- A young man of 18 was newly diagnosed with type 1 diabetes. He came to see me just prior to beginning injected insulin therapy. He was in what is called the "honeymoon phase." The honeymoon phase is basically the last gasping breath of the islet cells of the pancreas working to produce insulin. It is during this time where I have had the highest success of reversal of this condition. Again, I saw it in his eyes, he knew he would beat it, he BELIEVED he would beat it—and he did. He did not use any medications, only Superfoods and a few other alternative medicine additions.

Both of these patients, years later, are disease free!

Dean Ornish, M.D., demonstrates that lifestyle change affects one's gene expression.[23] His group found that stress management, improved nutrition, walking, and social support changed the expression of over 500 genes in men with prostate cancer. They also discovered that the genes which are associated with breast cancer and prostate cancer, and genes that cause heart disease, inflammation and oxidative stress (which causes inflammation), were turned off while protective genes were turned on.[23]

In another study, they showed that these same lifestyle changes increased telomerase activity. Telomerase is an enzyme which lengthens telomeres, which are the ends of our chromosomes that perhaps have a role in how long we live—kind of like our biological clock.[24] They found that the enzyme (and thus telomere length) was increased by almost 30% over only three months! This most certainly suggests that not only do these interventions prevent and reverse disease, but that they also have great potential to extend life span. Science aside—it makes perfect common sense: manage

A Note from Dr. Todd:

Set your intention. BELIEVE!

stress, improve nutrition, exercise, and be social as these will enhance your longevity and vitality.

SUPERFOODS AND THE SECRETS OF LONG LIFE

To recap, The China Study and a variety of other research, including my own, shows that if one changes their diet, they will drastically lower the incidence of disease. Period! I have found remarkable support of this across the cultures I have studied for greater than the past decade. In one recent study, Secrets of Long Life: Cross-Cultural Explorations in Sustainably Enhancing Vitality and Promoting Longevity via Elders' Practice Wisdom,[25] my research team and I explored study sites of the Eastern Afromontane and Albertine Rift region of Ethiopia, Africa; the Maya Mountains region of Belize, Central America; the Western Ghats region of India; and the Appalachian Mountains region of the United States. Our goal was to learn lessons from our longest-lived elders of long-existing cultures about how to be well.

Elders and elders'-elders, including a considerable cohort of centenarians (thirty-seven elders ranging from 65-106, and of these participants, 14 were verified centenarians), participated in this exhaustive study over a period of approximately 5 years. We grouped their Secrets of Long Life into three categories: philosophy and outlook, lifestyle, and dietary and nutritional practices.

These elders demonstrate that through a relatively comprehensive but simple set of practices we can enhance our vitality and promote longevity in sustainable fashion. Those principles are:

A Note from Dr. Todd:

The Secrets of Long Life
are NOT secrets!

- **Be positive**. They speak to, and demonstrate, the benefits of being optimistic. Adding life to years rather than adding years to life is the goal to which most strive—being active and engaged in the present provides for the future.

- **You are not just your body**. They illustrate the importance and ease of obtaining balance through considering health from a holistic construct, consisting of mental, physical and spiritual health and the necessity of the health of our natural and social worlds in nurturing our healthful balance.

- **Roll with it**. They demonstrate the importance of mindfulness (through meditation or purposeful activity or inactivity!), stress minimization, and respecting one's elders. They appreciate and welcome the cycles of life and the events of the life course—with resilience. They actively observe and partake in cosmic cycles: up with sun up, down with sun down, and they appreciate and are active with the change of seasons and our interdependence with the natural order and cosmos. Further, they demonstrate the necessity of honoring one's body through these changes, e.g., wear a sweater in spring despite how warm it may seem.

- **Get off the couch**. They demonstrate the need for regular physical and mental exercise, and importantly, the need for copious time spent outside observing and partaking in our divine physical, mental and spiritual interrelations with nature and cosmos.

- **Know yourself, and nurture your needs**. They teach that we must learn of our passion and purpose no matter how insignificant to others and act on these.

- **Eat well**. Through their diet and nutritional practices, they demonstrate that many of our disease burdens could be resolved through sunshine, pure water, and Superfoods. On topic, they also advocate for consuming food slowly and in meditation and moderation; chewing well and not diluting solids with liquids; not sleeping right after meals; and regular fasting and cleansing.

Since we are talking mostly about foods as you Eat Yourself Super, let's focus there (—but it is all related on the Superfoods journey!). We found a consistency among the diets of these elders: low amounts of, if any, refined sugar, white flour, trans fat, and a rich concentration of Superfoods which, by nature, have healthfully balanced sugars and fats. We absolutely know that Superfoods can begin prevention and reversal of the diseases of civilization. What do I mean by Superfoods?

Drumroll, please.

Here it is: Superfoods are plant-based, nutrient-dense, calorie-sparse, health-empowering foods.

These are the basis for the publication which you hold in your hands.

You see, for the first time in our history, people are eating plenty but starving. The SAD is full of nutrient-sparse, calorie-dense foods. This is against what the body needs to function, so the body says, "Continue to eat!" because it doesn't have the nutrients it needs, and satiation is not reached. This is why people can eat three pounds of pizza but not three pounds of broccoli. You get full with food that has food in it!

The practices I witnessed when studying cultures with significant longevity and vitality bring us back to the roots of our health. Superfoods diets, lots of pure water, sunshine, and taking part in that which brings us simple joy; be it our friends and family, walks in nature, time to meditate and relax, time to laugh and express feelings, or all of these.

Basically, we need to hit the reset button on our physiology if we are unwell! As I have discussed, we can do that with Superfoods and regain the balance or homeostasis that our health depends upon. Homeostasis is essential for life. Of course, there are a host of complicated factors affecting homeostasis in the human body, including oxygen and carbon dioxide concentrations, pH which is a measure of acidity or alkalinity in the body, salt and electrolyte concentrations, blood glucose and fat concentrations, nutrient and waste product concentrations, intracellular and extracellular volume and pressure, body temperature, fluids, gradients and chemical environments in and around cell bodies.

A Note from Dr. Todd:

Eat Yourself Super with Superfoods: plant-based, nutrient-dense, calorie-sparse, health-empowering foods.

Our greater than one hundred trillion cells are a social network coalesced into multiple communities or organs. These consist of types of cells with specialized functions. For example, red blood cells, approximately 25 trillion of them in your body, specialize in transportation of oxygen. This organ works with the community of lung cells which make up the lung and specialize in the gas exchange (oxygen in and carbon dioxide out). Our alveoli (functional units in our lungs) operate opposite of the plant world (carbon dioxide in and oxygen out). In a broader sense, we exist in a symbiosis with the plant world. Homeostasis consists of multiple dynamic equilibrium scenarios in our bodies and with our environment. Adjustment and regulation of these equilibria by the internal body systems and external environmental systems is necessary for good health—this adjustment and regulation is affected by your food.

A BIT OF BIOCHEMISTRY (JUST A BIT, I PROMISE)

Let's briefly discuss some of the requirements for human health in order to understand how the shift away from the practices of our longest-lived elders and our ancestors profoundly affects us.

We need carbohydrates, fats and proteins. We also need vitamins, minerals, trace minerals, hormone precursors, antioxidants, plant pigments and other phytochemicals. We even need biophotons as well as a multitude of other things that science has yet to uncover. All of this and then some we get from Superfoods and the optimal physiologic environment they spawn for the development of healthful symbioses (for example, gut flora which help us extract nutrients from our food, support our immune system, detoxify, and even synthesize some of our essential vitamins for us). We need these things for our metabolic processes that on the most fundamental level require energy exchange (energy which originally came from the sun).

The process of metabolism, though complex, can actually be broken down into two main processes: building up or anabolism, and breaking down or catabolism. In anabolism, our bodies combine useful energy with simple precursors to yield complex molecules. For example, the body builds Heme molecules to carry oxygen to our tissues and also turns carbohydrates (or sugars) into fats to store some energy for later. In catabolism, our bodies break fuel (carbohydrates, fat, and even proteins) down to yield carbon dioxide, water and energy—energy which we use for our processes. For example, with this energy we perform mechanical work (contracting muscle and cellular movements), the active transport of molecules and ions (necessary to move things against their concentration gradients), and the aforementioned process of catabolism.

In talking about energy in metabolism, for the most part, we discuss it in terms of heat or heat liberated. This is a Calorie. The heat liberated from 1 gram (gm) of carbohydrate or protein is about 4 Calories whereas 1 gm of fat is about 9 Calories. The energy breakdown available in foods consumed in the SAD approaches 40% (or more!) from fat, 45% from carbohydrates (much from refined white sugar), and 15% from proteins. Compare this to our ancestral diets, still observed by much of the traditional world (which includes our elders in my <u>Secrets of Long Life</u> research), their diets are roughly 15%-20% energy from combined fats and proteins—the remaining came from unrefined carbohydrates—this is the Superfoods diet. Our longest-lived elders eat as our ancestors have done—and we need to do. This level of Superfoods intake enables consumption of sufficient amounts of vitamins, minerals and trace minerals in addition to all of the other goodies necessary for longevity and vital living amidst physiologically appropriate levels of sugars and other carbohydrates, fats, proteins and their associated calories. All of this occurs in the context of an active lifestyle—they eat carbohydrates and burn their fuel. Importantly, this plant-based, nutrient-dense, calorie-sparse, health-empowering diet also effects an important physiologic balance which promotes optimal mutually beneficial relationships with our environment both external (think plant world; fields, forests and foodstuff) and internal (think microbial world; gut flora and microbiota of our bodies).

Science is just now beginning to demonstrate the wisdom of our elders and ancestors. Suffice it to say, for our purposes, that a Superfoods diet, rich in carbohydrates interspersed with adequate essential fats and balanced proteins, derives most of its energy requirements from carbohydrates and a smaller amount from fats and proteins. This diet is relatively protein sparing (this is important as protein catabolism negatively affects our blood vessels—it feeds into arterial disease and endothelial dysfunction) and exercises our biochemical machinery in the manner for which it is meant while providing a plethora of beneficial vitamins, minerals and aforementioned plant goodies necessary for optimal health. In short, as demonstrated by our longest-lived elders, this is our optimal nourishment status as humans. It promotes ease for our physiologies maintaining that ever so important homeostasis, or stable internal environment in context of our environment and challenges of life. For example, the maintenance of optimal ranges for pH, temperature, hydration, and ion concentrations in all the right places is easier done with this type of dietary intake. Going away from this causes problems with the equilibrium of the body.

This incredibly complex process of metabolism—and indeed, life itself—is dependent on an enormously complex variety of biochemical reactions. Nearly every single one of these reactions is mediated by its very own enzyme which basically turns this into that (in reactions that either require or liberate energy). Many enzymes need some help from cofactors though. View these cofactors as elements or minerals (which we have to take in through our food and drink), such as zinc, or coenzymes which are more complex organic molecules—many vitamins are coenzyme precursors (we have to take these in through our food and drink as well).

Major elements in our diet include: oxygen, carbon, hydrogen, nitrogen, calcium, phosphorus, potassium, sulfur, sodium, chloride, phosphorus, iron, iodine, magnesium, cobalt, copper, chromium, selenium, boron, molybdenum, manganese, and zinc. There are others too, such as, vanadium and lithium. In essence, these elements ultimately come into us from the air we breath (oxygen), the water we drink (oxygen and hydrogen) and the plants we eat (they get it all from the air, water, and soil). My family has a popular saying, "the soil becomes you." It really does via the plants. If you were to eat local Superfoods year-round and nothing else, and then take a sample of your soil and a sample of your hair, you would see that if your soil is low in selenium, you would be too.

The vitamins in our diets which serve as coenzyme precursors are commonly known as "water soluble vitamins" and include: biotin, cobalamin (vitamin B12), folic acid, nicotinamide, pantothenate, pyridoxine (vitamin B6), riboflavin (vitamin B2), thiamine (vitamin B1), and ascorbic acid (vitamin C). In contrast, vitamins commonly referred to as "fat soluble vitamins" are not coenzyme precursors and include: vitamin D (hormone activated from endogenous cholesterol and dietary ergosterol), vitamin A (hormone activated from dietary carotenoids), vitamin K (synthesized by healthfully balanced gut flora, but also in diet including green leaves), and vitamin E (several related plant-derived compounds exhibit vitamin E activity, there isn't a specific vitamin E though). These are all required for good health, but we have additional requirements, too. They take the form of essential fatty acids, essential amino acids, and a multitude of other things including plant pigments and the like. These are all part of the Superfoods diet.

To help you understand how to best consume a diet of Superfoods, I have created <u>Dr. Todd's Superfoods Pyramid</u> (Figure 5)—an easy guide to use as you <u>Eat Yourself Super</u>. By following the guidelines as you plan, shop, and prepare meals, you'll easily integrate Superfoods onto your daily plate. Superfoods also demand a complementary lifestyle as outlined by the <u>Secrets of Long Life:</u> mindfulness and mindful consumption, activity, time in nature, spirituality, social connections and paying attention to what your body needs are all part of the big picture.

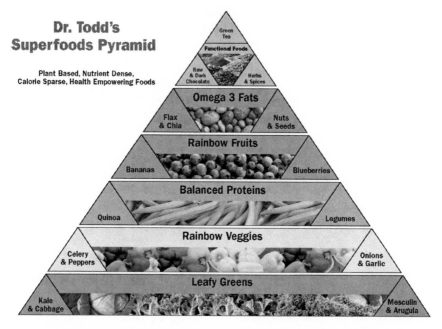

Figure 5. Eat Yourself Super with Dr. Todd's Superfoods Pyramid

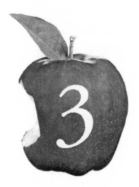

FOOD IN YOUR FOOD

So without further ado, let's address this delicious food. We now know we can promote bodily equilibrium through whole, real foods. What are "whole foods"? These are food items which have not been processed or refined, or if they had been, then only minimally so as to closely retain their natural state and nutrient spectra. The closer they are to the way they come out of the ground the better! Additionally, when possible, they should be consumed fresh and raw, and they should be local, organic, additive-free and non-genetically modified—just good old nutrient-dense whole foods as Mother Nature had intended.

A Note from Dr. Todd:

Don't eat petrochemicals, they are bad for you. They disrupt your endocrine system, cause cancer, and accelerate aging among many other things.

HARMONY IN WHOLE FOODS

These foods have a complex role in our bodies. Many phytonutrients have not been isolated and named (or even discovered), yet our bodies, in this perfect relationship we have with the planet that nurtures us, need these substances to be healthy. Taking a "greens pill" or a "garlic pill" will not have the same effect as eating raw, fresh greens or garlic. Similarly, taking a whole foods vitamin C tablet is not as useful to the body as eating a fresh orange or a serving of strawberries.

Health is not about analyzing the minute nutritional component of one single food and isolating it to promote wellness. It is about eating a variety of foods in their natural forms, or as close to them as possible, and knowing that you are consuming essential nutrients, and also compounds and energies not yet discovered—miraculous complementary systems of nature that work in concert in the body to allow health and vitality throughout your entire life. That is what a healthful, varied diet can do.

Michael Pollan's In Defense of Food discusses this throughout the book, and Campbell's China Study relates,

> "It's not that [nutrients] aren't important. They are—but only when consumed as food…Isolating nutrients and trying to get benefits equal to those of whole foods reveals an ignorance of how nutrition operates in the body." (pg 229)

For example, as we mentioned before, in fruit, sugars and fiber work together to slow sugar absorption into the bloodstream. In other foods, certain vitamins are concentrated together to provide the body with the greatest benefits. In other words, there is no substitute for home-prepared, close-to-nature, whole foods. I'm taking you a step further by encouraging consumption of Superfoods. The focus should be on the plant-based, nutrient-dense, calorie-sparse foods that our bodies need.

In addition, avoid as many animal products as possible. The vast majority of major publications regarding disease prevention and reversal support this, and in the healthiest parts of the world, animal (whether it flies, swims, runs, jumps or slithers) and dairy consumption is nowhere near the epic proportions reached in the Western diet. Eliminate animals and animal products from your diet for optimal health.

The Superfoods eating pattern represents a return to the lessons of our longest-lived elders who eat as our ancestors before us; a link to our roots—the places from which we come, the families in which we dwell, and the Earth to which we all belong. Sure, our ancestors hunted—they ate what they could, when they had to—but try running after a rabbit and then running after some leaves or tree nuts and figure on which they filled their bellies for the most part. In the northeastern United States, a considerable part of the diet was American Chestnut and other tree-nuts, add to that the greens in warm months and roots in cold, and that's the majority. The science is again very clear: low-fat, plant-based diet is key to optimal health. And, not only is the Superfoods diet naturally low in fat, but it effects intake of healthful ratios of essential fats and sugars—just as nature had intended. What this comes down to is balance—just what we need for our health.

A Note from Dr. Todd:

As evidenced by our longest-lived elders, the latest scientific research, and clinical practice in disease prevention and reversal, the Superfoods diet, and accompanying lifestyle, is key to optimal health.

MEALS ARE A SACRED PRACTICE

Meals the world over have unifying themes. People cook local foods, sometimes ones they grow themselves. Families gather around the table (or wherever the meal is taken). There is benefit to this ritual, to being close enough to what you eat that you understand what is in it, and to consuming it slowly and in a joyful, social situation. The seasonings, herbs, spices, and combinations in meals complement each other and human health. The sacred ritual of food is one which involves not only sustenance, but lots of the other good stuff as well—sensation, sensuality, mood, mindfulness, presence, elation, giving, gratitude and love to name a few. My family and I are of the mindset that when you love people, feed them. But only yummy, healthful food!

There is a reason the smell of a good meal is hard to resist! Aromatic herbs and spices have been used since time immemorial as an important part of our sensual, culinary and cultural worlds—and these awesomely flavorful herbs and spices also oftentimes have powerful medicinal properties which not only make them more valuable as foods, but the act of preparing and sharing food becomes a gesture of connection and healing and thus adds to the enjoyment of human experience and community. Sometimes elaborate feasts are consumed if there is a festive occasion, but even during these times, cultures with longevity eat real, whole foods that are carefully prepared—often with the same rituals as generations before. There is a sacrosanct quality to taking something into your body to nourish it. Treat the foods you eat with the respect they deserve. One of my favorite mealtime rituals involves sitting with food in front of me. I like to tell my children that there is no better test of patience than sitting down, hungry, with your plate in front of you (I learned that one in India!). I inhale the smell of the meal and allow myself to take a moment to salivate a little, in anticipation of the food.

What's actually happening here? I am beginning the digestive process by allowing saliva to enter the mouth; the salivary glands are excreting enzymes to allow my body to fully process the foods I eat—in particular, salivary amylase and lipase, which help to digest sugars and fats respectively. In addition, I recommend starting meals with bitter greens—this promotes the production of the correct digestive enzymes in the stomach.

SHOPPING GUIDELINES: WHAT THE HECK TO BUY

When you purchase food, the best strategies involve these steps:

- **Shop the perimeter as much as possible.** The highly processed foods tend to be found in the middle aisles of the grocery store.

- **Shop local.** This is becoming a food renaissance, of a sort, as communities rediscover their local farmer's bounty. We visit our local market so often that we are now friends with our favorite growers and we get some great foods set aside for us, as well as some great conversation!

As we discuss the eating practices of those cultures and individuals who display longevity as a rule, it is worthwhile to note that their foods are locally produced whenever possible and grown in rich soils. Your sense of place is in your local ecosystem. Your local ecology functions on a multitude of levels. Think of it this way. Let's say you plant a tomato plant in your yard, and you harvest the tomatoes and save some of the seeds. If you plant those seeds next year, your crop will do well—in fact, better than a crop grown from seeds purchased at the store. That's because the plant will be uniquely suited to excellence in that area. The ground ecology, light patterns, water availability, etc. are all exactly what that plant—reared in that region—needs to thrive. Your human body is similar. We are all indigenous—dig your roots in your region! The body is uniquely suited to consume foods grown locally. Look for other foods that grow in your region during that specific time of year. Around here, in Ohio, we have the forest bounty in spring starting with maple sap, then alliums: garlic and ramps, followed by a veritable explosion of other forest goodies. We have oodles of delicious spring greens. And, we have strawberries in June followed by cherries, blueberries, blackberries, raspberries and many more. Shortly thereafter we are moving into a bonanza of greens, fall harvest and then more forest goodies including various mushrooms and Paw-Paw.

A Note from Dr. Todd:

My fall pick! Black Walnuts are a wonderful runner-up, but my girls and I love Paw-Paw eating! Paw-Paw, *Asimina triloba*, is an understory tree species native to Appalachia. It is one of North America's largest tree fruits. It is in the Annonaceae or Custard Apple Family and has a number of tropical cousins. Being an understory tree, it starts out growing under the protective canopies of larger trees that like more sunshine. The Paw-Paw is super-nutritious eaten fresh off the tree or chilled as a desert. It is also a plant medicine used for a number of common ailments including constipation. Interestingly, the seeds, leaves and bark contain potentially useful anticancer acetogenins, but they are potentially toxic as well—so you eat the fruit and spit the seeds out.

Appalachian Ohio is home to the largest and most yummy wild Paw-Paw patches! We even have a festival honoring this delicious, local Superfood. As the Ohio Paw-Paw Festival group says: "Come wander the hills and discover why George Washington's favorite dessert was chilled Paw-Paw."

Root vegetables, squashes and cruciferous veggies are common during the late fall and early winter months, whereas apples, pears, and pumpkins are abundant a bit earlier in fall along with sequential harvests in late summer (tomatoes, corn, peppers, and basil—talk about nutritious and delicious!). Many fine foods grocers feature local products; I encourage you to try them. If you are lucky enough to live in an area with a farmer's market, that is an excellent place to shop as well! You will not only support your health, but your local economy, too!

Something miraculous happens during the seasonal cycles of the planet—our species is provided with chances to detoxify and fortify at transitions, grow and flourish at times of abundance, and at other times we become introspective, conserving energy and reflecting on that which is closest to us. Think of it: wintertime. It's colder, so we seek shelter, and find more time to look within. We sleep more as daylight hours become shorter. Our bodies need less energy. This is not an accident; our ancestors had access to fewer resources. This protective cycle allows the body to thrive given such change. Once spring begins to dawn, the maple sap runs—a sign that life is waking. Our elders taught me to welcome this change and drink this healthful sugary miracle with great joy! The first greens to show up on the forest floor are alliums: first garlic, then wild leeks or ramps. We consume, just as our ancestors before us, these beautiful signs of spring in mass quantities, and by doing so give the body a nice detoxification to start the local growing season. These alliums are among the first spring ephemerals or plants who spring forth and flower on the forest floor (sometimes for just a few short weeks) just prior to the trees' leaves coming in. They are soon joined by some of the other spring cleaners including "blood purifiers" and "reducers" represented by varied spring greens chock full of revitalizing, detoxifying phytochemicals and antioxidants, mild liver detoxifying laxatives and mild kidney cleansing diuretics—ramps and dandelions are among my spring favorites.

My girls and I rejoice in the spring and one of our main celebrations is ramp eating in the woods. A couple of baked home grown or organic potatoes (do NOT eat non-organic potatoes) or sweet potatoes make a fantastic complement to the ramp shoots and leaves right from the ground—a great break for a long spring hike in the woods! They are also amazing in salads. I so enjoy throwing a dinner party with a ramp centerpiece dressing where everyone LOVES it, yet no one gets what's in it, no matter how sophisticated the palate! On dandelions, I love the greens and crowns—the crowns sit atop the taproot and these succulent morsels are a true springtime treat. You can eat the greens right from the ground or in your favorite salad—the crowns are a delectable delight either raw, or lightly sautéed with aforementioned allium bulbs. Just be sure you are not eating dandelions that have been sprayed by poison. This practice has always puzzled me—people poison their lawns in the hopes of getting rid of dandelions, then they go to the store and buy them for their salads. Odd indeed and not good for people or planet—only good business for grocery stores and the chemical industry.

In addition, the closer your food is to the original source, the better the nutritional quality. This is because foods can be allowed to ripen on the tree, vine, or shrub because they are sold so close to their harvest date—not so with something shipped across the country—or world. This item must be picked before it is ripe to avoid rotting during shipment.

- Eat organics, whenever possible; at the very least, follow the guidelines for the "Dirty Dozen" (Table 1) and "Clean Fifteen" (Table 2).

The intricate cycles of life depend on a healthy ecosystem. Organic farming practices support this tenet—healthful soil spawns healthful food. When local produce (organic local should be your first choice) is not available, look for certified organic produce. Let me be clear—organic does not equal healthy, all of the time. It means, quite simply, that the food has been produced without synthetic herbicides, pesticides, fungicides, chemicals, petrochemicals, or genetically modified organisms (GMO's). They cannot contain or be processed with chemical additives, industrial food solvents or irradiation either. While this is an excellent step, they can still contain sugars, fats, refined cereal grains, and other items which we consume in overabundance or frankly, we should not consume period—read ALL labels. However, in our discussion, organics are a superior choice to conventional products—no doubt since they are more nutritious, more delicious and they are better for our environment and us.

I find it striking that organic produce requires a special label and certification, when conventionally grown, genetically modified foods do not. They can contain harsh soil additives, herbicides, pesticides and the like, which damage our health, yet no label is necessary. These oftentimes contain petrochemicals which clearly function as endocrine disruptors in the body (should we eat something meant to withstand multiple applications of weed killer?). This leads to a variety of ill health effects, such as inflammation, neurological dysfunction, cancer, etc. Not only is buying organic good for the planet, it is, unquestionably, better for your health. Organics allow avoidance of harmful chemicals, but the foods are also more nutritious. An apple is not an apple. Food grown in rich, organic soil, without the use of synthetic chemicals fertilizers, grows food with a more complete nutritional profile. As soils are depleted, the nutritional quality of food overall has declined; buying and consuming organics encourages repletion and responsible farming practices.

The Dirty Dozen represents those foods that show the highest concentrations of pesticides (some tested positive for as many as 67 different chemicals) after washing. As a general rule, avoid conventional produce if you are going to consume the entire item, or the skin.

Dirty Dozen:
Foods to Buy Organic

1. apples	7. grapes, imported
2. celery	8. sweet bell peppers
3. strawberries	9. potatoes
4. peaches	10. blueberries, domestic
5. spinach	11. lettuce
6. nectarines, imported	12. kale/collard greens

Table 1. Dirty Dozen: Foods to Buy Organic

Source: Environmental Working Group, http://www.ewg.org/foodnews/
summary/ Accessed October 14, 2011. Copyright © Environmental
Working Group, www.ewg.org. Reprinted with permission.

The Clean Fifteen showed little to no chemical residues once cleaned. These may still be genetically modified organisms or lack nutritional value though.

Clean Fifteen:
Foods with lower concentrations of chemicals

1. onions	9. cantaloupe, domestic
2. sweet corn	10. kiwi
3. pineapple	11. cabbage
4. avocado	12. watermelon
5. asparagus	13. sweet potatoes
6. sweet peas	14. grapefruit
7. mangoes	15. mushrooms
8. eggplant	

Table 2. Clean Fifteen: Foods with lower concentrations of chemicals.
Source: Environmental Working Group, http://www.ewg.org/foodnews/
summary/ Accessed October 14, 2011. Copyright © Environmental
Working Group, www.ewg.org. Reprinted with permission.

- If you must eat animals and their products, eat those that start with a healthy animal.

"Americans' appetite for meat and dairy – billions of pounds a year from billions of animals – takes a toll on our health, the environment, climate and animal welfare. Producing all this meat and dairy requires large amounts of pesticides, chemical fertilizer, fuel, feed and water. It also generates greenhouse gases and large amounts of toxic manure and wastewater that pollute groundwater, rivers, streams and, ultimately, the ocean. In addition, eating large quantities of beef and processed meats increases your exposure to toxins and is linked to higher rates of health problems, including heart disease, cancer and obesity."

— Kari Hamershlag, Environmental Watch Group
Senior Analyst, 2011 Meat Eater's Guide

Aside from significant environmental degradation involved with the manufacture of animals and their products, the scientific literature regarding their impact on human health is irrefutable: a low-fat, plant-based diet is the unquestionable gold standard. Animal products and associated excessive fat and protein consumption are harmful to the health (add to that excessive sugar and you have SAD), so, eating habits completely void of animal products promote optimal health.

If you must eat those things, weigh the benefits, and choose wisely—it all factors into your health equation. If you eat eggs make sure they are organic and free-range, also eat Superfoods with them. We love potatoes, peppers, kale, and mushrooms lightly sautéed up in the morning—try that instead of or with your occasional organic eggs. Eggs should be local, if possible, or organic, free-range, brown eggs. Cheese should be very carefully chosen as well and should be complemented with Superfoods if included in your diet. I tell people to avoid cow's milk by substituting nut milks like unsweetened almond, hemp, hazelnut and the like… they taste great. Also, nut milk's are very easy to make, see the Appendix for directions.

Remember, cows, pigs, chickens, fish and whatever else that are not properly cared for are not healthy animals. They are exposed to antibiotics, hormones, and toxins. In turn, by consuming these animals, individuals are not making good dietary choices. If meat is your preference, on the occasions it is consumed, look for wild game or organic, grass-fed, free-range, pasture-raised products, and prepare them at home with your Superfoods.

- I realize this is not about shopping, but it pertains here! Go easy on yourself. Baby steps are key! You have GOT to meet yourself where you are willing to be met.

First, start by adding more Superfoods to your diet. Then you can start to eliminate that which you should avoid—you will have more energy and willpower from the simple addition of more Superfoods in step 1. Whatever you do, do not overwhelm yourself—you will run the risk of giving up. Be sure to involve your family and friends too—tell them about your successes. Talk daily! And, changing your environment is also key to changing your patterns and your ultimate success (throw out the potato chips and replace them with kale chips and sprouted flax crackers. Yes. They are yummy. I promise). Always remember, as one wise elder said "everything in moderation—including moderation." It is perfectly fine to treat yourself—only try to go for the healthful raw chocolate and organic strawberries rather than the bowl of ice cream.

You know yourself. Are you one who wants to throw all the junk out of your house and shop from Dr. Todd's Superfoods Pyramid as some do, or are you one who wants to gradually phase in the Superfoods and then phase out some or of all of the processed, unwholesome foods? Only you know. Remember, the Superfoods diet is ideal for health as it is a plant-based, nutrient-rich, calorie-sparse, diet containing healthful ratios of sugars and fats and therefore it is health empowering combined with optimal hydration, sensible sunshine and active lifestyle—just as our longest-lived elders and ancestors teach. We have moved away from their practices and the pendulum is swinging back! If you are not already on a plant-based diet, consuming Superfoods with every meal, and a green tea aficionado who loves the outdoors, it is important to take steps toward making positive changes that are appropriate for you. This ensures success!

So I implore you, be realistic: a salad with each meal. Kale and other greens in your favorite soups and tomato sauces. Be sure to look for grass-fed/free-range organic meat and cheese and free-range hens' eggs when including animal products in your diet (but make no mistake animal products in your diet are not optimal). Try a plant-based meal several times a week (start with one, then two, then three....). By making incremental change, you will see incremental benefit. I find that my patients who attempt a massive, immediate overhaul have difficulty sticking with their good habits. Oftentimes, it is easiest to add a few things first rather than take away in the beginning.

A WORD ABOUT SUGARS

Since we are on the topic of what to buy, allow me to give you a crash course on sugar. The chemistry of sugars is relatively simple. There are monosaccharides, or single sugar molecules. The common ones involved in human nutrition are glucose, fructose and galactose. There are also disaccharides which consist of two monosaccharides linked. Three important disaccharides are sucrose (glucose linked to fructose—this is the common table or cane sugar), lactose (glucose linked to galactose—this is in milk), and maltose (glucose linked to glucose—this is the least common in food occurring in some germinating grains but it is an important intermediary in the digestion of complex carbohydrates). There are also polysaccharides, which mean many sugar molecules linked together, dietary polysaccharides include complex carbohydrates which consist of starch (which is digested into glucose) and fiber (which is not digested, but has a very important role mentioned following).

After all that gibberish, I will now make it simple. All of the above are carbohydrates. For the most part, only three carbohydrates make up the bulk of the healthful human diet: sucrose, starch, and fiber. In nature, we get our carbohydrates from fruits and veggies where they occur predominantly in disaccharide and polysaccharide forms as sucrose and complex carbohydrates (starch). For the most part, the body cannot absorb any of these as they are. The body absorbs principally monosaccharides, so, during the digestive process one's physiology must unhook the sugar monomers from the sugar polymer chains, whether they are two, as in the case of sucrose which is broken down into glucose and fructose, or many as in the case of complex carbohydrates, which are broken down to glucose.

Additionally, these are interwoven with lots of indigestible fiber (which incidentally is also a carbohydrate—but one we cannot digest and so from this point on I will refer to it as fiber), as well as other nutrients and beneficial phytonutrients.

The point is this: the final products of carbohydrate digestion in a healthful diet that contains far more starch than sucrose, consists of approximately eighty percent glucose (which is absorbed into the blood to be transported into cells via insulin) and roughly less than ten percent each of fructose and galactose amidst a sea of indigestible dietary fiber. This serves to slow digestion of the sucrose and starches and as a bottle brush or pipe cleaner binding toxins, metabolic byproducts, and the like from the intestines and depositing them in the toilet bowl, or woods, or wherever you happen to be.

This preponderance of glucose (in the form of predominantly starches) in our diet is precisely why our biochemical machinery is set up the way it is and why too much fructose (as in high fructose corn syrup) and too much sucrose (as in table sugar or cane sugar) are not good for us. The body can't send them on their way as nature intended. So keep this in mind as you shop: reduce hidden sugars and fats by paying attention and by eating your Superfoods which contain healthful proportions and rations of sugars and fats.

Many are probably familiar with the Glycemic Index (GI). The GI of a food relates how quickly the carbohydrates in that particular food raise the blood glucose levels. The higher the GI, the faster the glucose levels rise subsequent to eating (this corresponds to the speed with which your digestive machinery does its job in creating monosaccharides for absorption). Too much blood glucose is unhealthy as discussed prior. Eating a diet based on Superfoods limits the amount of high GI foods. For example, legumes (beans and their relatives), green leafy veggies (most veggies in fact), most fruits (berries in particular, pineapple and watermelon being exceptions), yams, sweet potatoes, wild and brown rice all have a low GI. Conversely, wheat (pasta is lower than bread due to the time it takes to digest pasta versus bread) pineapple, white potatoes, and some melons have a high GI (Table 3).

Notes on the Glycemic Index:

- Scale is from 1-100, with values 55 or below being low, 56-69 being medium, and above 70 high.

- These values should be considered approximations only as these foods have been tested under different conditions internationally.

- Values are calculated for foods that contain digestible carbohydrates. Foods that have negligible amounts of digestible carbohydrates do not have values. For example, most veggies do not have digestible carbohydrates therefore veggies like kale, collards, broccoli, and cauliflower do not have values. Similarly, a multitude of berries are loaded with fiber but very low in the digestible carbohydrates and therefore, do not have a value. Conversely, fruits that do have digestible carbohydrates have a value.

Glycemic Index (GI) of Common Foods

Bread: white, wheat and sprouted grain; 70, 70 and 55	Beans: kidney, soy, black and pinto; 20, 15, 30 and 33
Bread: pumpernickel and rye; 55 and 63	Lentils, 28
Corn, 60	Peas: chick, black eye and split; 36, 33, and 25
Barley, 22	Berries: blue and straw; 53 and 40
Quinoa, 53	Watermelon and Cantaloupe; 72 and 65
Rice: white and brown; 72 and 66	Apple, Banana and Orange; 44, 47 and 40
Rice: basmati and wild; 57 and 57	Potato: sweet and white; 44 and 69
Oats and Buckwheat; 57 and 49	Carrot, 16

Table 3. Glycemic Index (GI) of Common Foods.
Source: Glycemic Index Foundation, http://www.glycemicindex.com/ Accessed October 26, 2011.

SUNSHINE: THE BEGINNING FOR PLANTS AND PEOPLE

In modern society, there is an ever-growing disconnection from the natural world. This is worrisome because it is a false dichotomy—we are a constituent in nature and as such are inextricably intertwined with and dependent upon nature for our wellbeing. Two illustrations are our mutually beneficial symbiosis with the plant world and our reliance upon the sun.

As you may know, we exhale carbon dioxide and inhale oxygen while plants do the opposite in perfect harmony—but this is just the beginning. Plants need three main things to make their own food: give them a bit of sunlight, water and carbon, and the process of photosynthesis "captures" the energy of the sun in chemical bonds as sugars, which we rely upon, since this is what ultimately fuels our bodies. Once we have metabolized these sugars we return our waste to the earth and the cycle continues as our metabolic end products serve as beginnings to plants.

In addition to the aforementioned carbon and oxygen, we rely on plants for other essentials such as nitrogen and minerals. These elements are made more available to us by plants. Plants, quite literally, pull a great deal of their being from the air: carbon, oxygen, nitrogen and some water—sprinkle some sunshine, and voila! As you walk through the forest it is a marvel to realize that most of the biomass is actually accumulated from the air by these miraculous beings. The soil provides symbiotic organisms (which help out), minerals and trace minerals and more water. Plants make these minerals more available to us as well. Our physiologies are not very good at absorbing straight up minerals; they need to be "chelated" or bound to something that our bodies are good at absorbing (this works in reverse too—keep this in mind for cleansing and detox). Plants take these minerals in from the soil and chelate them. We eat the plants and absorb the chelated, bioavailable minerals. We also get all the other goodies that plants make in the form of phytochemicals which include vitamins and hormone precursors, antioxidants and pigments, and a slew of other biologically active compounds— many of which have yet to be discovered or even fathomed. Given this interconnected system of life on earth, it should not be a surprise that these plant products are absolutely essential to human life. We free their carbon-stored energy into our systems with the digestion of the plant as we metabolize their sugars produced through photosynthesis—their harmony with the sun—this is our intake of carbon, we get it from the plants.

The sun is the supreme source of energy for life on our planet. Without it, we couldn't exist. Yet, many people run and hide from the sun. In reality, moderate exposure is required for good health. You see, just as the plants photosynthesize, so too do we—but we make crucial hormones rather than sugars.

A major benefit of the sun has to do with the body's production of the "sunshine vitamin" or vitamin D. D is not actually a vitamin, but better described as a hormone. Vitamins are taken in through food whereas hormones are made internally. We are not designed to get our D from food. Rather, we are designed to make it within. Dietary concentrations of D, in nature, are relatively minute—it is basically not in food.

However, of note, a precursor is present in relevant concentrations in fungi or mushrooms. This is a part of the reason why certain mushrooms are an essential component of the Superfoods diet. In healthful balance, we take in fungi which provide ergosterol (this is the mushrooms version of cholesterol) and on a healthful diet; we make our cholesterol inside of us, principally in the liver. Cholesterol, being the father of all hormones, is made into a precursor molecule called 7-dehydrocholesterol, which is activated along with ergosterol to vitamin D3 and vitamin D2 respectively when ultraviolet B radiation (which is blocked by clouds, clothing, glass, smog and sunscreen) from good old sunshine hits our skin. Vitamin D3 (cholecalciferol) and vitamin D2 (ergocalciferol) are both inactive though and are further metabolized into 25-hydroxy vitamin D in the liver, and 1,25-hydroxy vitamin D in the kidney—this one is the active form which quickly serves its physiologic function—a steroid hormone in the sense that it regulates the expression of genes (recall the environmental component to epigenetics!), lots of crucially important ones.

VITAMIN D AND YOUR HEALTH

There is a growing consensus that there are widespread and overlooked D deficiencies among the general population, and the more we learn about it, the more problematic the situation seems. I have found in my clinical practice that it is a rarity to find someone above deficient levels, so one of the first things I do for my patients is to therapeutically replenish the D in their body. It is commonplace for vitamin D levels to register somewhere in the range which, for adults, is indicative of osteomalacia or, for children, rickets. Osteomalacia may manifest as diffuse aches and pain, muscle weakness, and weak, brittle bones. In essence, this is early osteopenia and osteoporosis which are due to lack of mineralization of calcium and phosphorus—the building blocks of our bones. Calcium and phosphorus come from our food, but it is D that is necessary to absorb these essential minerals from food in our digestive tract.

The current prevailing recommendations for vitamin D intake are woefully inadequate. First of all, it is clear based on the practices of our ancestors that we get D principally from the sun, and secondarily from our food. In today's world we are outside a lot less than our ancestors and when we are outside, we have a lot more clothes on. One solution is to lose the clothes and spend more time outside as generations before us have done. Another solution is a combination of dietary supplementation and responsible sun exposure.

Through my Secrets of Long Life research, the elders demonstrate the need to spend lots of time outside. This practice brings a multitude of benefits in health and wellness through stress reduction, spirituality, rejuvenation, meditation, and exercise to name a few. It also brings a slew of hidden benefits as well including immune system support and photosynthesis of vitamin D. Additionally, the elders point out the tremendous importance of balance, a meaningful note in this context given the fact that the dose of sunlight required for adequate D synthesis is less than the dose which brings on sunburn. Sunlight exposure can be part of healthful lifestyle inclusive of physiologically necessary D synthesis in context of reasonable photoprotective practices. This translates to roughly 20-30 minutes (which is approximately the minimum erythemal dose and effects the production of about 25,000 IU vitamin D3) outside in the sun as close to daily as possible—just enough time to turn the exposed skin pink and not burn it. And how beautiful is nature: during the winter months in the northern hemisphere, it is cold outside, but less exposure is necessary because the sun is actually closer to the earth. That's right, our closest point to the sun, or perihelion, occurs in the dead of winter—seasons are due to the tilt of the earth's axis—so we can get our D fix! Thanks, Mother Nature!

Unfortunately, nowadays people avoid the sun because of fear of skin cancer and premature aging. These fears are propagated by misinformation and exaggeration originating with doctors, media and interested business who stand to gain from selling you sunscreens, skin lotions and the like. Don't buy into it. If you cannot eat it, don't put it on your skin—it goes into your body just the same. Do not put petrochemicals on your skin—they are toxic!

A Note from Dr. Todd:

Watch everything you use as a personal care product! The only things my family will put on skin and hair are nut butters and oils. Specifically, raw, cold-pressed coconut oil or cacao butter, and beeswax lip balm. While you are at it, make sure you look at your soaps as well—the only soap we use is plant-based castile soap. My personal favorite is Dr. Bronner's Magic Soap. I love peppermint, it tingles the body and leaves one uplifted thanks to the rejuvenating, stimulating properties of peppermint oil. Peppermint is antimicrobial too and leaves you deeply clean without the toxic garbage common in so many other products.

In my view, the problems occur not with sun exposure, but with the aforementioned toxic petrochemicals on one's skin coupled with extremes in exposure. Our bodies do not do well with rapid transitions. We must ease into transitions.

Don't run outside without a sweater on in the springtime when it feels a lot warmer than it is, just as you cannot spend a majority of your time in the office and then walk outside one day, take the shirt off and lay in the midday sun for a few hours. It all has to do with slow transitions—honor your body. If you are about to experience an extreme shift in sun exposure as in the case of travel or something of the sort; cover up, spend time in shade, and if you use a sunscreen for you or your family, be sure that it is not chock full of petrochemicals and other toxins.

Millions of people are dying from lack of sun exposure—literally, about one million per year. I find it horrifying when new patients come to my practice after having suffered through an unsuccessful gamut of medical treatments for various ailments which are precipitated by a lack of sunshine—yet these patients' doctors, oftentimes, have not even checked their D levels! This happens quite often. With optimized D levels, emerging scientific literature suggests apparent risk reductions of roughly:

- greater than seventy percent for cancers across the board

- greater than eighty percent for breast cancer

- greater than sixty percent diabetes type 1 (recall this is the auto-immune type)

- greater than fifty percent multiple sclerosis

- greater than thirty percent of heart attacks, and the list goes on

These statistics are pored over and rapidly changing in the peer-reviewed literature. But, the science is clear and we need D. These data are not being given the consideration they deserve by mainstream conventional medical practitioners. Checking and optimizing one's D level should be at the top of EVERY treatment protocol.

In addition to healthful sun exposure in context of reasonable photoprotective practices, I routinely recommend that adults take vitamin D 5000 IU orally per day and for children it is usually less than this and based on age and weight. However, this is a maintenance routine and, as such, is only adequate once optimal levels have been achieved.

In my practice, I recommend my patients aim for an absolute minimum level of 60 nanograms (ng)/milliliter (ml). This is the goal, assessed by a blood test for 25-hydroxy vitamin D (the gold standard test) as well as keeping an eye on blood calcium levels as you don't want these too high. Keep in mind, when considering the raging debate and trepidation with regard to D repletion and D toxicity that the major side effects of D toxicity have to do with elevated blood calcium levels. Further, it is a physiologic fact that tremendous changes in D intake have little effect on the final quantity of 1,25-hydroxy vitamin D (the active form) that is formed—basically this means that your body uses the inactive D2 or D3 that it needs by activating them in the liver and then kidney. This is then used up, what isn't needed is not activated, rather it is not turned into 1,25-hydroxy vitamin D. When the blood calcium is high, the 25-hydroxy vitamin D is turned into a different compound with almost no vitamin D activity. In other words, it skips the last step and does not become activated. This is why people who spend a lot of time in the sun do not get vitamin D toxicity. Thus with therapeutic megadoses one is simply supplying the raw materials for the body to do what it needs. Importantly, considering thousands of patient encounters, I have yet to see any side effects (except for feeling great and disease reversal) to D repletion and I routinely use megadoses—literally—oftentimes in the range of a million or more IU's to optimize levels. Additionally, I carefully assess how my patients are feeling through the repletion process while using these megadoses to optimize levels as quickly as possible and then I settle into the aforementioned maintenance regime. Once optimized and on maintenance regime, checking levels annually is sufficient.

My patients, on getting their first megadose (roughly half a million IU's via an intramuscular injection of D3 (which will bring levels up approximately 10-15 ng/ml) many need two to three doses to become optimized), more often than not report vast improvements in health and wellbeing including improved energy, mental clarity, heightened senses including vision, better sleep and dream recall, weight loss, and decreased aches and pains just to name a few. Further, a multitude of pathologies cease to exist for them—from inflammatory conditions and all they bring, to more specific diagnoses like high blood pressure, you name it—D helps. If there is anything you take from this book, in addition to eat more Superfoods, please do drink pure water and have your doctor check your D periodically and then supplement and maintain an optimal level. There is a division of opinion on what optimal levels are; how low is too low and how high is too high are being hotly debated at present. However, as the years go on, I have noticed the prevailing views getting closer and closer to what I have been recommending and implementing in my practice for years now. The basis of my recommendations come from "stoss" therapy commonly practiced in European countries, in particular Germany. Indeed, stoss is the German word for bump, as in to bump up one's D level with megadoses of D.

D essentially helps make us who we are; it is responsible for our basic functioning with roles in prevention and memory, cognition, sleep and immunity. As mentioned, it is one of the first things I measure for when I have a new patient in my practice. When the deficiency is corrected, patients often comment that they feel "like a new person"—and it's no wonder! D is crucial, as is the sun. It is responsible for the epigenetic regulation of a significant component of your genome. Remember, genes cannot turn themselves on or off—we need our environment to do this and one way in which it does so is via sunshine and D. We know that in addition to the classic bone strength and health benefits (in other words, the prevention of brittle, weak bones or osteoporosis), this hormone has also been linked to the prevention of various cancers, diabetes type 1 and type 2, hypertension, chronic pain and multiple sclerosis; it modulates neuromuscular and immune function, reduces inflammation, and supports the very cell cycle (reproduction and rejuvenation of our cells—without which nothing could exist). Additionally, D helps support the immune system in fighting off infections, so the next time you are thinking about immune system support through cold and flu season, be sure your D is optimal. Also, ensure adequate intake of other fat soluble vitamins (A, E and K) easily done on a Superfoods diet. Vitamin A in particular as the A and D work together, in this regard.

So what does all of this mean to our Superfoods lifestyle? Go outside. Every day. Don't run from the sun. We need it. There is absolutely no question whatsoever that the sun exerts incredibly positive influence on our health and wellness in a multitude of ways including those which science does not yet comprehend. These benefits far outweigh the risk associated with sensible sun exposure.

YOU ARE PART OF THE ENVIRONMENT!

I mentioned that D is just one reason why we as a culture need to step outside more. Spending time outdoors holds a myriad of other benefits as well. As a modern population, we have become disconnected from the natural world. Despite this disconnection, we are very much a part of the natural world, and we are dependent upon it, whether or not we realize it. One look at classical poetry books will show anyone that nature has been calming and inspiring the human mind for millennia!

Studies have shown that those who spend more time surrounded by nature are less depressed, confused, anxious, and experience a surge in energy and vitality. In addition, visiting natural spaces such as parks and forests lowers stress levels and boosts immunity. Another example of a perfectly interconnected system! Exposure to plants and trees—which release oxygen and other compounds including phytoncydes which actually support our immune systems, the organic compounds which keep them healthy—is simply good for us; also it nurtures the delicate balance of systems. People the world over actually forest-bathe (or spend time in the forest) to breath in phytoncydes—you should too.

Human intimacy with nature has evolved cultures that have complex thoughts and practices involving the relationship with nature and its gentle, sustainable exploitation (think cosmocentric worldview and cultures which strive to live sustainably). This contrasts with the "modern" capitalistic orientation to nature—exploitation for profit no matter what the consequences (think another strip mall where there used to be a marsh or forest land). As we are seeing more and more often, this type of practice is dangerous for Earth and all of its inhabitants—us!

Spending time outdoors increases our sense of oneness with the Earth. That mind and body are distinct is a falsehood; if one is unhealthy the other often follows—nurturing both is essential. Time among the trees with the dirt beneath our feet is a time-honored way to do this. We were not meant to spend our days inside a building or surrounded by concrete, so when we do, it is reflected in our moods and in our health. Step outside and enjoy the beauty of nature to appreciate the world from which we come and fill up that spiritual reservoir for the days when it is most needed.

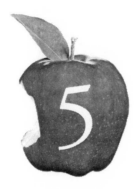

EARTH JUICE

Approximately fifty to seventy percent of your total body weight is comprised of water. Total body water is divided into two main parts. About forty percent is intracellular and about twenty percent is extracellular. Of our extracellular water, around seventy-five percent is predominantly surrounding and bathing our cells in what is called the interstitial space, while the remaining roughly twenty-five percent is contained in the blood plasma. This intracellular fluid, interestingly, has an electrolyte composition similar to ancient seawater! I think it is safe to say our bodies depend on water. And yet...

Here's a common conversation in my office:

Dr. Todd: You need to drink more water.

Patient: I don't like water. How do I make it more palatable? (Sometimes this takes an even darker turn as the patient utters the ominous "I hate water." All kidding aside, I hear this day in and day out from all sorts of individuals.)

Dr. Todd: [emphatically]: You probably have not had decent water enough to know that you love it—it is your life blood. Drink more pure water. You must.

And it is true. However, I am not surprised they "don't like water." The water that they have developed a sincere distaste for is tap water, specifically all of the noxious toxins contained in tap water. Tap water with all of its toxic contents is literally nauseating to many people and in particular to those who are in touch with their health or sensitive to such things. Their distaste for this contaminated water is likely a protective mechanism subtly driving them to find pure water. I never drink the stuff. Neither do my children—pure water comes from the earth, not the tap. Tap water is toxic. Not only should you not drink it unfiltered, but you should also not wash, bathe, or shower in unfiltered tap water if at all possible.

WHAT'S IN YOUR WATER

There is a modern problem with the contents of tap water: pollutants. These pollutants include: microorganisms, disinfectants, disinfection byproducts, inorganic chemicals, heavy metals, organic chemicals, radionuclides, and pharmaceuticals—both prescription and over the counter medications, hormones, and antidepressants—and industrial toxin run-off. These have been found in physiologically significant, even pathologically—or disease causing—concentrations in tap water. Pharmaceutical levels in city water are currently unregulated—any amount is legal! Chlorine is added to kill microorganisms, yet chlorine and its byproducts are poisonous to you. Most water has added fluoride—a caustic neurotoxin.

A Note from Dr. Todd:

It is horrifying that toxic byproducts of industry are added to our water under the auspices of dental hygiene. I have never used fluoride and I have no cavities. Don't buy into the bold-faced lies. A family sized tube of toothpaste with fluoride has enough fluoride to poison, possibly fatally, a small child! Avoid fluoride for your health and the health of your family. Many in the United States don't realize how unnecessary and dangerous this is—in fact, most European countries refuse to fluoridate the water supply because it has not been deemed safe—as mentioned along with the other halogens, it is an endocrine disruptor, and is linked to problems in the central nervous system, skeletal system, and in the kidneys.

This rampant disdain for water is promulgated by the nature of the toxic sludge that comes from your tap and it is aided and abetted by the beverage industry and poor regulatory governance which allows water to be violated and toxins to be added to our water supply. People turn from the tap and pop open a tab or bottle-top. Bottled water is no better. In fact, it is worse. The bottled water industry has obvious issues with authenticity, transparency and even purity. Much of the bottled water on the market at present is simply tap water with the added plastics which letch from the bottles into the water you are meant to be drinking. Bottled water is not good for you nor is it good for our environment. Not only is it less regulated, and therefore oftentimes has more contaminants than tap water, but studies have shown that it loses to tap water in terms of taste as well. This is a horrifying reality with deleterious effects toward global health and wellness. Here is my advice to you all—connect to your water just as you connect to your food on your Superfoods journey. The more of us who demand pure water, the better for us all, particularly our children.

Spring water, or "Earth Juice," as my family has been fond of calling it for generations, is a miraculous substance, the properties of which have continued to not only give life, but also enrapture many for millennia. (Want evidence? Put any child in the water and you have an instantly happy kid!) I realize this is not a discourse on water, but there are some pertinent things I would like to share. I was raised with and maintain a deep reverence for water, sun, moon and indeed all of nature and the cosmos. I can tell you that I view water very differently than most based on the things that I know and see.

Scientifically, water is very complex and it seems that the more science uncovers about water, the more questions arise. For example, there is wonderful work being spearheaded by Professor Gerald Pollack of the University of Washington, Seattle. He is revolutionizing scientific understanding of water with work that has profound implications for all of science and indeed all of life! His book Cells, Gels and the Engines of Life (Ebner and Sons Publishing, Seattle, Washington, US) has been noted as a preface to the future of biology. Essentially, he demonstrates that in addition to the well known three phases of water (gas, liquid, solid) that there is an extensive fourth phase as well which occurs at interfaces. In stark contrast to current reductionist views, which consider water as a mere background carrier of the molecules of life, Pollack has shown that water is a central player in life. In other words, it isn't just a solution—there is a lot more to it. Some of the miraculous properties of water are related to its remarkable internal cohesion. Basically, water sticks together—this is why it has a high boiling point; why bugs can walk along on the surface of water; why clouds form, and so on. This internal cohesion is enabled at least in part by the fact that water molecules ($H2O$) form hydrogen bonds with other water molecules. The substance maintains a rapidly fluctuating, hydrogen bonded molecular structure; it is an orderly structure that moves. In other words, water is a liquid crystal. Albert Szent-Gyorgyi (born 1893-1986), commonly referenced as the father of modern biochemistry, was awarded the Nobel Prize for discovering vitamin C said, "Life is water dancing to the tune of solids."

Victor Shauberger (born 1885-1958) was an Austrian forester and a scholar of nature and water. He was a proponent of learning from and then working with nature as opposed to working against it. He developed water theories involving energy, vortices and multiple dimensions of flowing water. His theories note that nature creates vortices to promote balance and that flowing water, in essence, rejuvenates itself through vortices, bubbles and like natural processes. His tremendous insight, inspired solely by the study of nature (he refused to go to college as he thought it would inhibit his ability to learn from nature) was correct in a multitude of respects based on newly emerging science—but also common sense and intuition if one were to let it guide them. Once again, science is showing what traditions have known for millennia. We must work with nature, not against her.

DRINK TO THIS

So, all of this said, naturally flowing, gravity-fed spring water is best for us—this water is ripe for picking. It is alive with energy that has been enabling life since life began. And, as for the vortices, well, just ask any shaman of any tradition and they will tell you how important they are.

My family has been going to a local spring to fill our water containers for three generations; prior to that, the spring was in our back yard. It is a ritual in health and something that I recall with great fondness. Just as I went to the "water place" as a child, so too do I go now as a father with my children. It is an easy and fun regular expedition: "Who wants to go get water?" "We do!" As of this writing, my children are seven and four, and I have not given them water from the tap. They know that pure water comes from the earth.

When I was a child, we visited a gravity-fed, never-ending trickle down a moss-and-lichen lined shale and sandstone hillside within an Appalachian mountain holler. There was also a pipe sticking out of this verdant hillside in the middle of the woods to make it easier to fill jugs. We would visit the spring generally every Sunday as do we still to this day. Despite being continually admonished to stay clean and dry, my sister and I would inevitably end up soaked from head to toe from playing in the babbling stream that was fed by this spring—we were playing with all the water critters. All that playing worked up our thirst and our appetite. We would drink water right from the earth and gorge on watercress growing amidst this fertile oasis as we filled our containers and took in the forest and all associated energies. We never came home clean. Or dry. It was marvelous.

For those of you who think you don't like water, or think that drinking water is a chore, I ask simply that you try it just once as it comes from the earth. For many of you, this may well be all you need in your path to wellness—hydration! So, take a sip, just as generations before have done and after us all will do! I have yet to hear from one person who has done this and not reversed their opinion on water. In fact, most adopt water as their principal beverage immediately after their real water experience. This is how it should be. It is a different experience when it comes from the earth.

A Note from Dr. Todd:

Glass carboys and containers work best for water—sometimes the five gallon ones are a bit too heavy to easily manage; the one or three-gallon carboys are my recommendation. If you must use plastic, stay away from recycling numbers 3, 6, and 7, and avoid Bisphenol A (BPA) and phthalates. Plastics are horrible for our health and the environment. They contain carcinogens and endocrine disruptors, among many other things.

I use glass carboys for a bunch of other things as well, for example, fermenting apple cider to make **hard cider**. Here's how I do it: fill a glass carboy up with raw apple cider (<u>has</u> to be raw), put a glass airlock on the mouth and watch and wait. That is it! No, you don't have to add yeast or anything else. It's all in there. You will see the carbon dioxide (fermentation byproduct) bubble through the airlock. This bubbling lasts typically a few weeks depending on the sugar content of the apples you use. After it stops bubbling, let the yeast settle a few days and then enjoy. Our ancestors have been imbibing in healthful fermented foods and beverages for millennia—enjoy them, guilt free, and in balanced fashion as a part of your Superfoods diet. The fermentation process provides a plethora of bioavailable vitamins in particular the B's—all that and it's chock full of nutritious yeast.

Remember, not only are you what you eat, you are what you drink! Drink living water ripe for health and rejuvenation.

Hydration is essential. Adipose tissue (also known simply as fat) has lower water content relative to other body tissues. As a consequence, the more fat tissue on a body, the less hydrated the body becomes. Women, then, tend to have a lower percent of their body weight as water because, relative to men, they have a higher percentage of adipose tissue. Obese individuals approach the extreme low end of the range. So these individuals may become dehydrated very quickly.

Dehydration is dangerous for anyone—and if you happen to have a body with a lesser concentration of water you have to exercise even more caution. Aside from the obvious sign of thirst and bright yellow urine, the dehydrated individual may experience headaches, fatigue, difficulty concentrating, weight retention, and even kidney stones. Well-hydrated bodies feel and function best; it is simply necessary to life processes.

Here is the rule: if you are not voiding light yellow to clear urine, then you need to drink more pure water (B vitamins aside, as they can turn your urine yellow). Be aware that while it is hard to drink too much water, it can happen in certain scenarios. One extreme condition that can develop is called hyponatremia, which is basically low serum sodium outside the cells caused by a relative excess of water or loss of sodium in the body—this could be for a variety of reasons, and occurs in such scenarios as athletics, imbalanced intake and/ or loss, and the like. This leads to water moving into and swelling the cells, which causes a problem in the brain in particular and causes confusion and more serious issues. Obviously, you want to avoid these extreme scenarios and others by balancing intakes of sodium and other minerals with water—a well hydrated, Superfoods diet does the trick. Dehydration, of which hypernatremia is an extreme example, is a decrease in total body water relative to sodium—it results in dehydrated and suboptimally functioning cells. Small drops in total body water drives the injurious effects of dehydration and include fatigue, digestive issues, dry skin, heartburn, constipation, premature aging, and issues with one's immune system (including both autoimmunity and weakened immune system) to name a few of the common ones.

You lose roughly a liter of water a day simply being inactive—this is called insensible loss—add to that all that you lose with activity. Don't wait until you are thirsty. Thirst is a primitive mechanism; by the time you are thirsty your total body water has already dipped considerably below optimal hydration. In short, you must drink lots of pure water. Optimally, I mean gravity-fed spring water— this is ripe and ready for drinking, similar to an apple on a tree. A distant second choice which many opt for due to convenience and logistics is combining reverse osmosis with an effective carbon filter in a filtered water system. Ground water or well water is oftentimes a good option too, but it depends on the quality and extraction processes among other things.

STEPS TO PURE WATER:

- Find a local spring. A good place to start is out in your community: go to any local farmers market and ask the organic growers. Alternatively, a good online spring database is www.findaspring.com

- Connect with and know your water. Spring water is usually best assessed onsite by a number of techniques, including such things as clarity, temperature, smell, taste, and common sense. A good strategy is to talk with those who are getting water there to determine the reputation of the spring. Oftentimes you will talk with individuals who have been drinking the water for years, or even generations. Also, if the art isn't enough and you want some science, there are a number of independent analytic laboratory testing groups who can test your water for you—this goes for ground and well water too.

- Tap water suppliers publish their data, so read these annual reports. A good online resource is Environmental Working Group's National Tap Water Atlas, you can type in your zip code and learn all about your tap water: www.ewg.org/tap-water

- If you must drink and cook with tap water, filter it (and change your filters). Choose a good filter that will remove contaminants from your water. The Environmental Working Group's Water Filter Buying Guide is a tremendous resource: www.ewg.org/tap-water/getwaterfilter

- The ideal would be reverse osmosis filtration combined with an effective carbon filter—this gets the gunk out. This is about the best option out there next to spring water. Also, remember to consume adequate minerals and remember water is nature so give your water some love, sunlight, and a vortex type stir prior to drinking. Give it a little sunshine, maybe five minutes or so—as mentioned, there is a lot to the ordering of water and approximating what is actually happening in nature to maximize our health benefits. In other words, do what your ancestors and longest-lived elders have done. Ok, enough water wizardry for now.

- Remember the young ones, expectant mothers, and elders. They need pure water too.

- Pass up bottled water for the spring or the filtered tap. Don't drink bottled water due to the plastics leeching and the obvious social irresponsibility of the whole bottled water thing.

- Remember to carry a stainless steel or glass bottle filled with spring or filtered water everywhere you go and drink up.

- Don't forget your washing, bathing and showering water—remember, it gets in you just the same. There are whole home filters or you can get shower and bath filters in addition to the filter for your drinking water.

A Note from Dr. Todd:

Reverse osmosis water is good in the sense that it filters out much of the nasty stuff, including fluoride. However, it is bad in the sense that it filters out much of the good stuff, like minerals, as well. If you routinely drink reverse osmosis water, do ensure adequate mineral intake, which a Superfoods diet does quite well. Additionally, you can add a pinch of mineral salt like Real Salt or Celtic Light Grey Sea Salt to your drinking water. Raw apple cider vinegar is an awesome source of bioavailable minerals as well. You can make a great **lemonade** with an organic lemon, a tablespoon of apple cider vinegar and a half tablespoon of grade B maple syrup to the gallon. Another yummy mineral and electrolyte trick is to intersperse your water with rejuvenating beverages like green juices. I love my Champion Juicer. One of my favorite juices is based on green apples, kale, celery, cucumber, ginger, garlic and a cayenne or jalapeno pepper (Yum, my mouth is watering as I write this). Celery is miraculous for electrolyte repletion, so is green coconut water. In fact, green coconut water has the same electrolyte concentrations as human plasma. I have hiked for days in the hot jungle to gratefully emerge to a few green coconuts!

Ok...now I have you drinking more pure water and spending time outside—maybe a garden or a daily walk? You are ready to get to the most delicious part of health: the Superfoods themselves.

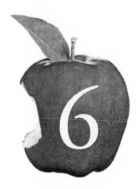

GREEN LEAVES:
THE MORE, THE MERRIER!

This book has grown not only out of my passion and purpose, but also my experience. As such, it has been focused by a multitude of successes witnessed as my patients, students, friends, family and community empower their health on the Superfoods journey. It works—I see it every day.

The journey varies depending on the person: same goal for all, but different paths and progress rates. This point bears repeating here: I have found that there is great merit in meeting people where they are willing to be met. The incorporation of a Superfoods diet, in my experience, must begin in a non-overwhelming fashion to ensure adherence and success. Be kind to yourself, honor your body and take baby steps if that is what you require.

Remember, the SAD is all around us and it is replete with garbage, including refined white flower and sugar, refined fats and trans fats, animal and animal products, etc. People have grown accustomed to eating these things in a multitude of ways, including as emotional comfort foods. Rather than saying "don't eat this" or "say goodbye to that," I start with the "add this" and "add that." The exclusionary beginning becomes overwhelming. Avoid the "what do I eat then??"

scenarios. If you ban everything you currently eat, you won't have any idea where to go from there! It is easy and effective to first start with some additional green leaves in your diet, then add a bit of this and a bit of that. This works as an excellent beginning point.

Once the additions begin (and stick), people experience the benefits of Superfoods through improved energy, mental clarity and well being. With improved energy and confidence the eliminations seem to happen naturally; people phase the no-no's out of their lives for good in whatever fashion they want. The cravings for the good stuff really seem to kick in and it becomes easy to live the Superfoods lifestyle.

So there you have it. Start by adding some green leaves!

I oftentimes say, "my patients, and those who seek this information, are geniuses." They are (Which, then, of course, makes you a genius)! These are the individuals who have critically analyzed the conventional system for one reason or the next and consequently have ended up sitting in front of me. They seek a more sustainable solution; they want to dig out the root cause and not just mask symptoms. Good holistic practice involves the resetting of the normal physiology to the best of one's ability—and sometimes it is a slow process. Patience is important, as is perseverance.

Now, on to the base of the Superfoods pyramid for excellent health: Green Leaves!

GREEN IS THE COLOR OF HEALTH

Your ancestors ate about six to seven pounds of green leaves per day in season. That's like a grocery bag full! This is the food that is most missing from the SAD. This is a shame, because your health is inextricably intertwined with these beautiful green leaves. As the availability of processed food has increased, we have, as a culture, been shifting away from eating leaves, veggies, fruits, nuts and seeds to the consumption of grains—cereal grains, and animals that eat cereal grains. This shift away from the traditional diets of our ancestors, no matter who you are, has not been without consequence. As mentioned, we are seeing increases of inflammatory diseases, arterial disease, diabetes, digestive problems, cancers, and even depression as a result of this change.

People the world over eat greens. I have eaten them the world over with them! Sadly, some of my favorites seem to be a one-time deal, but they illustrate an important point. People collect leaves from field and forest, and they then eat them. I can't understand why this seems to be so strange to some people! I have eaten all sorts of things, from mind-blowing (and even mind altering) curries from the rainforest to tangy delectable delicacies from mountainous highlands and other natural areas the world over, my backyard included. Oftentimes, the proportions, seasonality and specifics of the plant bounty vary and, for the most part, each culinary experience is unique.

Pollan's In Defense of Food discusses the Western dietary shift "from leaves to seeds" (pg 124). He states,

> "Put in the most basic terms, we're eating a lot more seeds and a lot fewer leaves, a tectonic dietary shift the full implications of which we are just now beginning to recognize…Leaves provide a host of critical nutrients a body can't get from a diet of refined seeds. There are antioxidants and phytochemicals; there is fiber; and then there are the essential omega-3 fatty acids found in leaves, which some researchers believe will turn out to the be the most critical missing nutrient of all."

He also discusses the harmful shift in ratio of omega-3's to omega-6's in the body as this occurs (and we'll talk about that more a little later).

A Note from Dr. Todd:

My eldest daughter Kaia's first food was kale (little Lily's was hot peppers—that is why she is so fiery!). She loves kale to this day and so do I. I am asked routinely how it is that my children eat so healthfully. My answer is simple—"my children eat what I eat." Our children see what we do and then do it—vice versa too in certain scenarios and if we are wise! If we praise greens via our culinary palate then they will too. Period. On many a day in Appalachia, I have filled my belly on Sassafras leaves, violets and other forest greens on long hikes in the woods. My children do the same. The sophistication of their palate for greens never ceases to amaze me. For example, recently we all went to Belize where I have been working with the Maya for over a decade. We sat down to many traditional meals hosted by dear friends in their palm-thatched huts from the jungle to seaside. After sampling the local, seasonal greens dish that kept being set before us one evening, the girls asked me "Daddy, what is this?" Kaia remarked something along the lines of, "it tastes like spinach, but isn't." I told her that she was absolutely correct. I told her that she was eating Callaloo, a local Amaranth—a Caribbean greens delicacy. The plot thickens though—I have eaten curried Amaranth in India and a salty but sweet Amaranth soup in the Andes. Guess I'll have to take her there next to reward her discerning taste buds! You see, Amaranthus, which is a genus of plants collectively known as Amaranth, is a vast mixture of plant species (more than 60) valued around the world for their leaves as veggies. I have eaten many of them referred to by a multitude of names including "Red Spinach," "Taro," our beloved Amaranth, and even the aforementioned Callaloo! She knew a good thing!

Remember this: pound for pound, calorie for calorie, these are the MOST nutritive Superfoods in existence. Leafy greens:

- are loaded with their green pigment, chlorophyll;

- are a rich source of bioavailable minerals (including iron, calcium, potassium, and magnesium);

- are a rich source of fat soluble vitamins, including K and E—rich in K and this is crucial, in particular in those with imbalanced bowel flora;

- are a rich source of water soluble vitamins, including C and many of the B vitamins, including folate, a B vitamin that helps reduce risk of birth defects;

- provide a variety of phytonutrients including beta-carotene, <u>lutein</u>, and zeaxanthin, which protect our cells from damage and our eyes from age-related problems, among many other effects;

- are essential for vascular/arterial health and contain phytonutrients which help with vascular relaxation.

As producers (aka, they make their own food…remember high school biology…), leafy greens are loaded with chlorophyll and bioavailable vitamins and minerals; they are highly alkalinizing and detoxifying. Chlorophyll fights the diseases of civilization with its antioxidant and anti-inflammatory properties, and it can reduce difficulties we typically associate with aging. Acids are produced as wastes from the body's metabolic processes. In homeostasis, our physiologies work to maintain a narrow pH in the alkaline range that is necessary for good health. Leafy greens are alkalinizing as are Superfoods in general.

Overall, they help the body not have to work as hard in keeping this balance. A healthful bodily blood pH is about 7.4 on the pH scale—it is kept there through the rich supply of physiologic buffers in body fluids. An acidic diet and composition can weaken the immune system and put the body at risk for inflammation, illness, and cancer. Those who avoid leafy greens can impinge on their body's natural cleansing and healing processes in other ways too. These veggies add fiber to the diet and act as an additional cleanser, like a brush from the mouth all the way through the digestive tract.

In addition to chlorophyll, alkalinization, and a high concentration of other nutrients, a real superstar present in greens is vitamin K. Recent research has provided evidence that this vitamin may be even more important than once thought (the current minimum RDA is likely grossly inadequate) and many people do not get enough of it since it is low in their diets and their bowel flora is off balance and not producing what it should in vitamin K.

What is this vitamin K? It is well known for some of its roles, less well known for others. These roles include:

- healthful blood clotting;

- helps protect bones from osteoporosis;

- helps prevent and possibly even reverse arterial disease/atherosclerosis by reducing calcium in arterial plaques;

- acting as a key modulator of healthful inflammation, and helps protect us from inflammatory diseases, including arthritis;

- may help prevent and/or reverse diabetes.

In order to reap the vitamin and mineral rich, alkalinizing, detoxifying benefits of these powerhouse Superfoods, you should consume a good amount of leafy greens each day. These should include the following <u>Green Leafy Superstars</u> as often as possible:

- **Kale**. This green contains massive amounts of phytonutrients, chlorophyll, vitamin K, indoles, lutein…the list goes on and on! Kale has been deemed a nutritional superstar over and over again.

There are many, many types of greens, some of which work better in lightly cooked dishes (don't kill your food by overcooking it), some better raw (since they are more tender).

Note from Dr. Todd:

Remember, cooking your food creates glycation products, which then drive diabetes. It also destroys life-giving enzymes, nutrients and the bioavailability of certain minerals. Try eating more raw foods by using such strategies as soaking, sprouting, dehydrating, and light steam sautéing foods. When you cook, do not overcook, and if you can cook it lightly and keep it under 118 degrees, this still constitutes "raw." I am not saying that you need to be completely raw, but you should eat an abundance of raw fruits and veggies, no doubt. Aim for seasonality, too: more raw in spring and summer, more lightly cooked and warming foods in fall and winter. This is how it should be for a healthful balance. In some instances, the bioavailability of certain nutrients improves with light cooking, for example, mushrooms and root veggies.

- **Cabbage**. Phytonutrients and sulfur compounds contained therein are very important for detoxification and maintaining vitality.

- **Mesculin** and **Arugula**. Great as salad or cooked lightly into pastas!

- **Cilantro** and **Parsley**. These are potent herbs that can spruce up a variety of dishes and help with detoxification and purification among other things.

- **Fermented greens** (and other fruits and veggies)—such as sauerkraut and kimchi. These provide a plethora of nutritional benefits grown through the fermentation process and include bioavailable B vitamins (much of these nutrients are destroyed by pasteurization or cooking), they support digestion and healthy bowel flora as well, and they even aid in detoxification. Humans have been drinking and eating fermented foods since time immemorial—so too do the longest-lived elders in my research. So go ahead and get yourself a traditional fermentation crock and do include them in your Superfoods diet.

I do realize that one hurdle some may face is that they aren't really sure what to do with all of these greens they should introduce into meals. There are countless ways to prepare them. Start with a huge salad with every meal—then eventually turn the salad into the meal.

Go for raw veggie juices, dehydrated kale chips, raw greens, whatever, whenever—throw them in stews, sauces, and even smoothies. You name it—they are good for it. You will learn to crave them because your body will (does) love them!

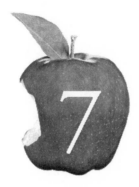

EAT THE RAINBOW (EVERY DAY)

Why eat the rainbow? The answer is simple... plant pigments. They are essential to your health! These different plant pigments have varying roles in the body and are necessary for balanced physiologic function. "What are plant pigments?" you may be asking yourself. They are plant compounds that are perceived to have a color. The major classes of plant pigments are: chlorophylls, anthocyanins, carotenoids, and the betalains.

As the chlorophylls and the carotenoids are the main photosynthetic pigments in plants, they are relatively ubiquitous. The chlorophylls appear green and serve to capture energy from the sun, and the carotenoids appear yellow-red and serve principally as antioxidants to the plant. They both exhibit antioxidant properties for us and chlorophyll has been shown to be a potent anti-inflammatory as well—this supplants the universality of traditional healing practices in using green leaves to treat inflammation. However, certain green leaves and plants are better for this than others due to the presence of additional phytochemicals.

This illustrates an important point: general activity and specific activity. Most photosynthesizing plants have general anti-inflammatory activity given their chlorophyll and other anti-inflammatory pigments and effectors (e.g., kale, broccoli), but some have more powerful anti-inflammatory activity and can be applied as more potent anti-inflammatory agents (e.g., turmeric, a spice we will talk about more in a bit).

Anthocyanins appear in a wide range of colors ranging from red-orange to blue-violet and serve principally as antioxidants to the plant. Anthocyanins, next to chlorophyll, are probably the most important plant pigment group for our health. Betalains appear red or yellow, and once again serve as antioxidants to the plant they call home. They replace anthocyanins in certain flowering plants.

MORE COLOR, GREATER BENEFITS

So, up the pyramid we go. Directly above our leafy greens base lie the rainbow veggie component of the pyramid and, two levels up since they should be consumed to a lesser degree, our rainbow fruits. Basically, you want to eat twice as many veggies as fruits.

In nature, that which is brightly colored is meant to attract—male birds, for example, as well as flowers, fresh fruits, and fresh vegetables. This variety of color in foods is not an accident or merely decoration. They are meant to attract for pollination or consumption for seed dispersal—this is how they propagate themselves. Plants ask us to eat their goods in this way. They also protect themselves from damage caused by ultraviolet and visible light. They need to be in the sun, just as we do. They protect themselves with these pigments—we protect ourselves by eating them. People who eat copious amounts of fruits and vegetables as part of a healthful diet protect their skin and reduce their risk of chronic diseases, including diabetes, arterial disease (which, as you know, leads to high blood pressure, heart attack and stroke), and some types of cancer.

Eating the rainbow, as our longest-lived elders suggest, provides the body with a diversity of plant pigments which protect our cells from damage. Studies continue to demonstrate beneficial effects of plant pigments, which include antioxidant, anti-inflammatory, anti-glycation (remember what drives diabetes complications), and anti-microbial. Further, they protect from cancer causing carcinogens, protect from cardiovascular damage and promote improved circulation, and even improve vision among many other effects. As if that isn't enough, they are also quite tasty!

Not only does the rainbow strategy provide one with the spectrum of plant pigments and antioxidants, but also the benefits of additional phytochemicals these plants bring (for example, the "indoles" a type of phytochemical in broccoli, cauliflower, cabbage, kale, and other cruciferous vegetables helps to protect against some types of cancer). They also provide a variety of phytonutrients in nutrient-dense, calorie-sparse Superfoods form! What else can boost the immune system, lower cholesterol, detoxify the body (different antioxidants promote the elimination/neutralizing of different oxidants—which cause damage), and may even slow the very aging process? Nothing.

Ok, ok. I know there is a bewilderingly complex array of plant pigments, antioxidants, phytochemicals etc. That's why I tell people to eat the rainbow: ROY G BIV. You do not have to know all the specifics. Trust me and let color be your guide, as our ancestors have done.

It is important to note that as Yin and Yang demonstrate quite well—the fabric of nature is balanced. Light and dark, hot and cold, up and down, front and back, the same holds true in our physiologies. Our physiologies are actually a series of oxidation and reduction reactions inextricably intertwined as electrons or charged particles (more accurately wave-particles…we are not really sure of their specifics…they are most certainly cosmic). These get passed back and forth in the process of life. My point is that we need oxidants and antioxidants to exist in balance in our bodies for health—when the scale is tipped in either direction, problems ensue. Given those toxicities we discussed earlier, it would seem we are increasingly bombarded with free radicals—which are oxidants. We need to balance with antioxidants. Why? T. Colin Campbell puts it nicely:

> "Free radicals are nasty. They can cause our tissues to become rigid and limited in their function…To a great extent, this is what aging is…But here's the kicker: we do not naturally build shield to protect ourselves against free radicals. As we are not plants, we do not carry out photosynthesis and therefore do not produce any of our own antioxidants. Fortunately the antioxidants in plants worn in our bodies the same way they work in plants. It is a wonderful harmony. The plants make the antioxidant shields, and at the same time make them look incredibly appealing with beautiful, appetizing colors. Then we animals, in turn, are attracted to the plants and eat them

and borrow their antioxidant shields for our own health. Whether you believe in God, evolution or just coincidence, you must admit that this is a beautiful, almost spiritual, example of nature's wisdom."

(The China Study, pg 93)

How can they perform these "fountain of youth" functions? By minimizing damage from free radicals that injure cells and damage DNA. Free radicals form a chain reaction in the body that can damage cells. These free radicals are highly reactive, unstable molecules that are missing an electron, so they look to bond with other molecules. Once they do, that molecule is now missing an electron, and the reaction continues. This is highly destructive to the body.

Antioxidants present in Superfoods, especially rainbow fruits and vegetables, take away the destructive power of free radicals by attaching to/neutralizing the molecule and stopping the chain reaction. By doing so, these compounds prevent and reverse some serious disease processes. Basically, we cannot live without plants if we want to thrive.

A Note from Dr. Todd:

I recall a particular meal that I had in the Western Ghats mountains region of Southern India. It illustrates a great point—in India, food is honored. It is eaten with one's hands. In Western culture we separate ourselves from our food with a piece of metal used to shovel it in. I was served a delectable array of curries, chutneys and rice on a banana leaf (not a plate)—the elders told me that the banana leaf being warmed by the food secretes certain things into the food. They said these help one's digestion. Anyway, the food was amazing and dazzled each taste and sensation on my palate in stark contrast but balanced fashion—a veritable symphony of tastes and sensations. The elders told me that we must balance the Six Rasas (or tastes—but more like experience and impact of food on eater) for good health. The Rasas are salty, sour, bitter, sweet, pungent or heat (e.g., peppers), and astringent or kind of, well, like tannic or mouth drying (e.g., lentils). I am no stranger to eating with my hands, as I pretty much always do this anyway—in particular greens and salads. There is something spectacular about the texture of food—both in the hand and mouth. Food prepared with love is extra yummy and when you love your food, you honor it. Feel it! Learn from the children. Ditch the flatware and eat some Superfoods with your hands. You use your index, middle and ring finger on your right hand to sort of scoop a bit and then kind of push it into your mouth with your thumb. Yum.

SO WHAT'S IN THE DAILY RAINBOW?
A FEW SPECIFICS!

- **Red:** Reds are commonly colored by plant pigments called lycopene (a carotenoid) or anthocyanins. Lycopene in tomatoes, watermelons, beets, and pink/red grapefruits helps to reduce risk of several types of cancer, in particular lung and prostate cancer.

- **Orange** and **Yellow:** Oranges and Yellows are colored principally by carotenoids—but there are other yellows, for example, certain betalains. Beta-carotene in sweet potatoes, pumpkins and carrots is converted to vitamin A (which is a hormone not a vitamin) that maintains healthy mucous membranes and healthy eyes. It works in concert with vitamin D at promoting a healthy you. Research has shown that plant-based carotenoids help reduce cancer risk whereas synthetic actually increases risk—this is the famed carrot study. More reason to get your nutrients from whole foods! New data is emerging on vitamin E that is suggestive of this same concept—synthetics are toxic!

- **Green:** Can't leave out those greens in a section about color! Greens (leafy and otherwise!) are colored green by chlorophyll. Chlorophyll is the supreme superstar nutrient as in addition to being an anti-inflammatory and antioxidant, it is deeply nourishing, detoxifying and alkalinizing—all integral to healthful physiology and the prevention of disease. Interesting side note: the leaves on deciduous trees appear green until the chlorophyll shuts down for the season, then the carotenoids show their colors. This is how we come to enjoy the fall foliage as we do! Green veggies and dark leafy greens like green peppers, peas, cucumber, celery and spinach contain lutein as well. Lutein works with another carotenoid called zeaxanthin, which is found in corn, red peppers, oranges, and grapes, and helps to keep the eyes healthy. Together, these phytochemicals reduce risk of cataracts and age-related macular degeneration, which can lead to blindness.

- **Purple:** Purples are colored by our beloved anthocyanins. For example, they abound in blueberries, blackberries (even some reds like strawberries, raspberries, and red grapes) and other fruits and vegetables which then act as powerful antioxidants which protect our cells from damage and promote healthful aging and heart health. In addition, they help reduce the risk of cancer, stroke and heart disease. <u>Blueberries</u>, especially, are a Superfoods superstar. A handful of blueberries a day works wonders. Even though they are sweet, they are actually anti-glycating—in other words, anti-diabetic! They are great on their own or mixed with sprouted wild rice, in a smoothie, or on a bowl of quinoa. Their season passes quickly, but they freeze well, so stock up when you see them at your farmer's market or on bushes that you planted in your yard.

Other fruits, such as acai, goji berries, and other international superstars, are often available. Be adventurous with your choices, but be sure to balance with sustainable local berries. <u>Rainbow Veggie Superstars:</u>

- **Onions**: These contain thiosulfinates, sulfides and sulfoxides, all of which are important for detoxification and the maintenance of vitality. Ramps, or wild onions, are awesome raw or in my famous ramp dressing. Play around with the preparation. Onions are extremely versatile.

- **Garlic**: Yum! Garlic contains allicin—this is more concentrated with greater surface area exposed and it is degenerated by heat. So chop it small or smash it and eat it raw. It is an important antimicrobial, and contains diallyl sulfides, which are important for detoxification and the maintenance of vitality. Eat as much raw, smashed garlic as you possibly can! It's delicious crushed up and mixed with apple cider vinegar as a dressing on greens.

- **Celery**: This is nature's electrolyte repletion—healthful salts! Don't drink sports drinks—eat more celery!

- **Peppers**: Another big favorite...lots of flavor! Capsaicin (in the spicy ones), lutein and zeaxanthin support healthful circulation and eye health. Hot peppers are a thermogenic superfood! Their heat actually speeds up your metabolism. Capsaicin has a multitude of health empowering effects including reduction of levels of substance P in one's body. This is crucially important since substance P is the physiologic compound that triggers inflammation and pain.

While eating red-hot peppers might well burn your tongue, they can cool aches and pains through the interruption of pain perceptions elsewhere in your body. This occurs via the capsaicin triggering the body's release of endorphins. Endorphins are produced by the pituitary and hypothalamus (endocrine or hormone master glands in the brain) in response to pain, exercise, excitement, arousal, love, orgasm and pepper eating! They resemble opiates (like morphine) in their physiologic action and in their ability to reduce perceptions of pain and promote feelings of wellbeing. Red-hot peppers also contain salicylates, like the willow, which is from where aspirin originates. All that goodness AND they are chock-full of vitamins, minerals and beneficial plant pigments, in particular the red ones.

The big idea is to go for a variety of colors—along with your greens, go for yellows, oranges, reds, purples, and the whites of cauliflower, garlic and onions. Enjoy the exploration and try different combinations of foods. There are such a myriad of ways to prepare and consume them—the sky is literally the limit! So eat up, and remember to eat twice as many veggies as fruits and enjoy the superstars.

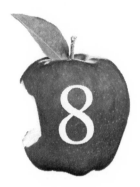

BALANCED PROTEINS: BUILDING BLOCKS

Plants—Our Protein Roots

Approximately three fourths of our body solids are comprised of proteins. Proteins are used structurally, as enzymes, as accompaniments to DNA, to contract muscle, and to carry oxygen, as well as for a multitude of other specific functions throughout the body. The properties that describe protein's diverse roles in our makeup are so complex that they constitute a major part of the field of biochemistry. Take my word for it…we do need proteins—and we get them in optimal fashion for health on our Superfoods diet.

But what exactly is a protein? Basically, proteins are functional strings of amino acids (the monomer unit of proteins) that assume a structure and function based on the properties of the individual monomers interacting with one another once they become strung together. Kind of like a string of beads, only some of which like one another. The ones who like one another coalesce and those who do not repulse; the end result is a unique structure with relevant function. Not only are amino acids used to form proteins, but they also function in other capacities, for example, as enzymes, to break down food, to grow and repair tissues, and a multitude of other functions.

Amino acids can be generally classified into three categories:

- Essential (ones we cannot make and so must get from our food)

    ♦ Threonine, Lysine, Methionine, Valine, Phenylalanine, Leucine, Isoleucine, Histidine, Tryptophan

- Conditional (ones which are usually nonessential, but are essential in certain scenarios including times of growth, illness or stress)

    ♦ Glutamine, Tyrosine, Glycine, Cysteine, Proline, Serine, Arginine

- Nonessential (ones we can make and so we do not need from our food)

    ♦ Alanine, Asparagine, Aspartic Acid, Glutamic Acid

You do not have to eat all essential and conditional amino acids at every meal, but a balanced diet throughout the day does the trick (In addition, be sure to ensure adequate intake of both essential and conditional amino acids in children and during times of illness and stress).

So back to the structure. These monomer amino acids are comprised of various atoms and are strung together by what is called a peptide bond or linkage—essentially a bond between a nitrogen atom, usually represented by an amino group and an acidic group on the amino acid monomers (The nitrogen is key here…see below). In this fashion, amino acids are literally the building blocks of life. So, as a consequence, they are in everything you eat—even green leaves. Not surprisingly, one of the best sources for these building blocks is a family of plants known as legumes, which include peas, beans, and lentils among others.

A Note from Dr. Todd:

Let's take a step back here and talk about nitrogen a bit. You need protein, and protein needs nitrogen—let's view it as a building block of a building block. The major reservoir of nitrogen is the atmosphere as nitrogen gas makes up the majority of our atmosphere. Most living things, however, cannot directly access this nitrogen—they need help. The process of atmospheric nitrogen being reduced to a usable form occurs via a process called nitrogen fixation. This is done principally by certain bacteria which, for the most part, live in symbiotic relationships on the roots of plants. The bacteria provide nitrogen to the plant, and the plant provides certain things to the bacteria. Why is this important to your Superfoods diet? Because these guys love legumes. That's why legumes are amazingly balanced proteins—they have plenty of nitrogen fixing going on in their roots via this symbiosis. This is why it is a common practice to rotate other crops alternately with legumes; the legumes fix nitrogen into the soil for the coming crop. The nitrogen flows from the atmosphere via the bacteria into the plant into you and then back into the earth in various forms to be assimilated along with additionally fixed nitrogen. This cycle—the nitrogen cycle— is necessary for life as we know it.

THE PROTEIN MYTH

There's a protein myth in Western culture. We're way too obsessed with protein. Yes, protein is an essential part of our diet as it provides these amino acids. But, on the SAD, the average person consumes greater than double the protein their body needs. Add to this the fact that the main sources of protein consumed on SAD tend to be animal products, which are, in addition to the other negatives we discussed earlier, high in fat. Most are surprised to learn that their protein needs are actually much less than what they have been unhealthfully consuming.

It is relatively easy to ensure adequate protein intake as long as the diet contains a variety of greens, vegetables, legumes and healthful whole grains. Plant-based proteins are a key component in the healthy body as they contain essential nitrogen packaged as amino acids, along with fiber and bioavailable vitamins and minerals. These are highly nutritive, alkalinizing and detoxifying, contain ZERO cholesterol (remember we make all that we need) and balanced fats in all the right places. Really: Popeye didn't walk around with a can of tuna, did he? No way. Spinach—a close sister to quinoa! And he was on to something: protein is abundant in leafy greens, veggies, and, the Balanced Proteins and their Superstars.

Quinoa (keen-whah)— a plant native to South America that has been consumed for millennia by the Inca and their predecessors, is a Balanced Proteins Superstar because of its high total protein content (~15%) and its awesome balance of essential amino acids and conditionally essential amino acids—it has them all in good amount and they are quite bioavailable! Quinoa is not a cereal grain as it is not a grass, nor is it a legume, but rather more closely related to spinach and beets. It is the seed of *Chenopodium quinoa*. It has a nutty quality, and is quite versatile. *Chenopodium* sp. or Goosefoot is widely distributed and in some circles it is viewed as a weed. Indeed, I grew up weeding an edible relative to quinoa right from our Appalachian garden—*Chenopodium album* or Lamb's Quarters is an awesome tasty green—kind of like spinach. This is the gardener's revenge—eat the weeds! Purslane is another of my favorite garden weeds—great in salad or just right from the ground as a midday snack. If you love your pasta, which has a lower GI than breads (due to its density), Quinoa pasta is an excellent alternative to white flour pasta.

Essential Amino Acid Composition in Quinoa	
Essential Amino Acid	**Quinoa, mg/g protein**
Methionine	18
Lysine	51
Tryptophan	15
Valine	39
Threonine	38
Phenylalanine	34
Histidine	24
Isoleucine	32
Leucine	79

Table 4. Essential Amino Acid Composition in Quinoa. Source: Ruales & Nair, Nutritional quality of the protein in quinoa

(*Chenopodium quinoa*, Willd) seeds. *Plant Foods for Human Nutrition* 42: 1-11, 1992.

BEANS, LEGUMES,
THE MAGICAL PROTEIN SOURCES

Legumes are unified by the characteristic pod that splits in two along seams on its sides—think of green beans. They are second only to cereal grains in providing agricultural food worldwide. In contrast to cereal grains, however, the seeds of legumes are rich in balanced proteins. There are thousands of legumes! Lentils, peas, chickpeas, mung beans, lima beans, soy beans, all kinds of beans…a multitude of seeds, all of which contain essential proteins.

Soaking and sprouting your legumes is a great way to enhance your Super-foods journey (see Appendix). Soaking simply refers to just that—soaking them to remove some of the harsh phytochemicals, including tannins, in the skin or seed coat (meant to protect the seed from being eaten and digested), which also eliminates bitterness. Soaking also softens the beans for consumption. Sprouting indicates actually beginning to grow the legume or seed.

Why sprout? Picture seeds (including legumes) as having a backpack of sugars and starches it carries along with it. These sugars are on hold in order to sup-port life, should conditions become favorable. When you sprout, the enzymes are made active, so that is why the sprouted seed is more bioavailable and healthier—less stored carbohydrates and more of these active enzymes which support life. And you can sprout just about anything with a seed coat! When I was a kid, there were always a bunch of large ball jars covered with cheesecloth next to the sink in the kitchen, sprouting radish seeds, mung beans, alfalfa seeds, you name it, pretty much all of the time.

The only thing you won't be able to sprout is something that has already come out of its seed coat, such as, for example, walnuts. They are quite versatile in the kitchen—you can add your sprouted legumes to soups (hot and cold), salads, dips, and spreads, or eat them simply as sprouts.

WHOLE GRAINS OR NO GRAINS

There are literally hundreds of thousands of plant species, many of which have edible fruits, shoots, roots, tubers, seeds, and/or leaves. Yet, approximately 17 spe-cies provide greater than 90% of humanity's food supply. Even more alarming is that of those 17 species, the vast majority comes from 4-5: wheat, corn, rice, bar-ley and soy. Excluding soy (which is a legume), these are all grasses (cereal grains). People on the SAD eat way too many of these! They are not eliminated from your Superfoods diet, however, they are to be included as Balanced Proteins (and there-fore must be whole grains not refined) here and there, NOT as carbohydrate filler!

Grains are plants cultivated for their edible grains, which are actually a type of fruit called a caryopsis. This is composed of three parts: the endosperm, germ, and bran. In their natural state, whole grains are a rich source of balanced proteins as well as bioavailable vitamins, minerals, carbohydrates and fats. However, with refining, there is removal of germ and bran and the remaining endosperm is mostly carbohydrate devoid of other fiber and nutrients. So go ahead eat these as a component of your balanced proteins, but be sure to go for the whole grains—remember, sprouted is best!

In addition to your legumes, chenopodium, and whole grains, be sure to include a diversity of nuts like almonds, Brazil nuts, coconuts, cashews, walnuts, hazelnuts, and pinenuts, as well as seeds like chia, flax, hemp, pumpkin, sesame, and sunflower seeds. Your Superfoods body will thank you!

A Note from Dr. Todd:

There are some delicious sprouted breads and tortillas readily available. For example, Food for Life's Ezekiel Bread and Tortillas are marvelous versions of sprouted grain products.

GET MOVING

If you are active (and I hope you are!), your body has a relatively increased need for balanced proteins. Activity is essential to good health! Side note here…you need daily exercise in the form of stretching and movement. Stretch often daily; just like the family cat or dog, first thing they do on waking is stretch! Go walking or hiking daily for an hour and a half. In addition to this, you need both resistance exercise (minimum of thirty minutes weekly), and aerobic exercise for twenty minutes or so three times a week (roughly 80% max heart rate).

Basically what this comes down to is that you have to use your body. Be active—try brisk walking or hiking, swimming, trail running, Yoga, or Tai Chi. Be creative and have fun! You can combine elements of the above (daily movement and stretching, resistance and aerobic) into single activities, too— such as Yoga and Tai Chi (plus you get the added benefit of daily meditation—which you need to do anyway). Be sure to mix it up and use your body, hang out in the woods a bit, and consume the right proteins!

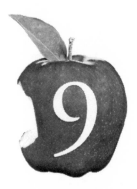

UNRAVELING OMEGAS

Walking up the pyramid past proteins and fruits, we come to fats—the good ones! As you may know, there are good fats and there are bad fats, but oftentimes, it is a matter of perspective or balance. The key to healthful fat intake is consuming the good or essential fatty acids—which you need—in balanced form and while eliminating the bad fat, which you do not need (but is all around us). Not rocket science! Remember, your ancestors knew they needed fat and so they sought this valuable substance out in nature. What they found though were healthful plant-based fats in predominantly healthfully balanced ratios and physiologically appropriate packages. This is not the case in today's world, where a multitude of fats (including man-hydrogenated (or trans) fats! Yuck!) are readily available. We must be very careful in seeking out healthy fats and minimizing, if not eliminating, bad fats in our culinary choices.

FATS IN A NUTSHELL

Pun intended. Fats from the nutshell are usually good for us, whereas artificially produced trans-fats should be eliminated completely. Saturated fats from animal products should also be eliminated, but interestingly, specific saturated fats—

from plants such as coconut are good. <u>There is no question with regard to the science: the best fats are plant fats consumed in their natural form as plants.</u> This is exactly how our ancestors and longest-lived elders get their daily fats.

These plant fats contain *essential fatty acids,* or EFA: so named because without them we cannot survive. We need to get them from our food since we cannot make them in our bodies. Modern science seems to know this; EFA are all the rage these days. You'll see them touted on food labels all over the place. The advice to consume EFA omega-3, -6, and -9 is currently everywhere—yet this is incorrect. For optimal health, you must eat more omega-3's and try to avoid overconsumption of omega-6's and omega-9's. Further, for the most part, they should be in food, not highly refined oil. If pressed out of the plant, these fats, or better referred to as oils (since most are liquid at room temperature), are unnaturally high concentrations of fats and Calories.

Basically, EFA are polyunsaturated fats, classified into the omega-3 (alpha-linolenic acid) and the omega-6 (linoleic acid) groups. Omega-9 is not considered "essential" because the body can manufacture it given the consumption of other unsaturated fats. It is important that the correct foods are eaten to ensure a balanced variety, and thus, optimal health. When these EFA are present in healthfully balanced amounts, the body uses them to build cell membranes, regulate inflammation and to support the brain, nervous system and the cardiovascular system among other things.

THE OMEGA CODE

First of all, the majority of the SAD is based on cereal grains, which are low in omega-3's. The consequence of this is chronic inflammation and illness, including cancer, as omega-3's are crucial to balancing the inflammation-inducing omega-6's—of which are in ample supply in cereal grains. The omega-6's are direct precursors to pro-inflammatory arachidonic acid. We need both inflammatory and anti-inflammatory functions in our body, but we need them in balance. Inflammation is how we fight off an infection or heal a wound, strain or sprain… you get the picture. The problem arises with imbalance. Our ancestors ate, and cultures with remarkable health patterns continue to maintain as demonstrated by our longest-lived elders, diets of approximately equal ratios of omega-3's to omega-6's.

Whereas our ancestors consumed approximately equal amounts (ratio of 1 to 1) of omega-3's to omega-6's, those following the SAD consume them at ratios of at least 1:10, but more likely 1:20. This "modern diet" has people walking around in perpetually pro-inflammatory states, which, as you'll recall, spawns diseases of civilization, including pathologies such as cancer. The good news is that this inflammation is reversible with Superfoods, in particular leafy greens and omega-3's consumption in context of a relative decrease in omega-6's. The bad news is that omega-6's are consumed in very large amounts in the SAD (they are hard to avoid) because the diet relies for the most part on a small number of cereal grains: corn, rice, barley, and wheat (I challenge you to read a handful of processed food labels and not see at least one of these on nearly all of them) all rich in omega-6's and low in omega-3's.

There are a multitude of edible plants out there—let's not focus so much on the cereal grains (or their oils!). Moderation is a good rule to live by in most areas of life, and food is no exception: it is not good practice to consume much of anything in overabundance. Eating four grains over and over is going to cause problems. In this case, it is because it leaves little room in the diet for other foods. In the SAD, this can be very plainly seen in the EFA consumption ratio. We, as a culture, even feed cereal grains to animals! The animals are walking around in perpetually pro-inflammatory states—not natural, not good for them, not good for you if you eat them, not good for the environment. They want to graze, but they are given grain. When they are consumed by people, the perpetual pro-inflammatory state continues.

Omega-3's are consumed in rich quantities on the Superfoods diet. The majority of these omega-3's are in the form of alpha-linolenic acid (ALA). There are longer chain omega-3's formed in the body as well—they are eicosapentaenoic acid (EPA) and docosahexaenoic acid (DHA). EPA and DHA are the more metabolically active forms of omega-3's, however, there is substantial evidence that each of these omega-3's has independent and substantive effects on cardiovascular health. We need them all.

The conversion of ALA to EPA and then DHA occurs as the body adds length to these fats starting with ALA. DHA is the longest. Basically, this occurs via a series of enzymatic steps involving, for the most part, enzymes called desaturase and elongase. There are a couple of things that facilitate the body's conversion of

ALA to longer chain EPA and DHA. These are a reduction in dietary omega-6's, since these compete with omega-3's for the desaturase enzymes, and, the adherence to a plant-based Superfoods diet since animal products, fish included, have been shown to slow the conversion of ALA to EPA and DHA. Populations on the SAD tend to rely on fish oil for their metabolically active omega-3's, but fish cannot produce EPA or DHA—they get it from eating algae. Since the fish supply is threatened (and one runs the risk of heavy metal toxins in fish and fish oil), you might be relieved to know that you can meet your requirements for ALA, EPA and DHA more optimally on the Superfoods diet while helping to preserve the fish supply!

A Note from Dr. Todd:

Preserve the fish—eat Superfoods instead! You can easily meet your requirements for ALA, EPA and DHA on the Superfoods diet. However, if you must eat fish, be sure it is wild, healthy and toxin free. Eat wild caught only…be sure it is a clean, organic, sustainable source, which really goes for any animal products you may consume. Be extra careful here though, since fish consumption exposes the body to environmental pollutants and heavy metals. Also, be aware that there are marketing ploys at play here—know your source.

WHY EAT OMEGA-3'S: EIGHT MAJOR REASONS

- A diet rich in omega-3's is cardioprotective and reduces the risk of arterial disease. People who eat copious amounts of omega-3's rich Superfoods are less likely to have high blood pressure, heart attack or stroke.

- Omega-3's protect from insulin resistance and diabetes.

- Omega-3's protect from oxidative stressors and cancer.

- Omega-3's are anti-inflammatory and necessary to balance the pro-inflammatory omega-6's.

- Omega-3's may improve mild symptoms of menopause, such as hot flashes and breast tenderness.

- Omega-3's are essential for eye, brain, and mental health.

- Omega-3's may also help with mental focus and clarity.

- Omega-3's may help protect against autoimmune conditions, arthritis, and pain.

Aside from our leafy greens and veggies foundation, which should include brussel sprouts, cabbage, broccoli, kale, spinach and a myriad of others that are rich in omega-3's, there are several other excellent sources that are easily obtained and work well in a wide variety of dishes.

MEET THE OMEGA-3'S SUPERSTARS:

- **Walnuts:** Brain food! They even look like little brains. Omega-3's are in oodles of other nuts and seeds as well. Be sure to try hemp seeds, and hemp and almond milk! Some of my favorites!

- **Flaxseeds:** Flaxseed is rich in ALA. Like most plant-based fats, flaxseed fat is an unsaturated fat that is healthy for the heart and cardio-vascular system.

- **Chia Seeds:** Chia is an edible seed that comes from *Salvia hispanica*, a member of the mint family that grows abundantly in deserts of southern Mexico. They have been consumed as a Superfood for millennia. They were a main component of the Aztec, and other indigenous peoples of the regions diets. They were given as survival rations to Aztec warriors. It is very rich in omega-3's, even more so than flax seed, and is also rich in antioxidants, fiber, calcium (more calcium than cow's milk), phosphorus, magnesium, manganese, copper, iron, molybdenum, niacin, and zinc. It stabilizes blood sugar as well and thus is a great Superfood for use in prevention and reversal of diabetes.

A Note from Dr. Todd:

Personally, I prefer chia to flax (but I love them both). Chia is advantageous over flax because, first, it has more antioxidants, so it has a longer shelf life. It is more bioavailable than flax, because flax needs to be ground to best be used by the body; this opens it up to oxidization and rancidity much more rapidly than whole-seed chia.

Chia tastes great on its own or in salad. You can sprinkle it into soups or whole grain dishes, or put them in baked goods. It forms a gel with water and makes an easy, nutritive energy food. My daughters like to call chia seeds soaked in water "frog's eggs", and I agree it does look a little like them! Like the super-athletic Tarahumara, an indigenous group in Mexico, who routinely run greater than 100 miles at a time on chia, my girls love to eat chia—and they keep on going! I cannot keep my children out of the Superfoods.

The Tarahumara and others make chia into a beverage called Chia Fresca—chia, water, lemon, and a little healthful sweetener, such as raw honey.

This beverage recipe reminds me of a story. It was spring of 1999 and it was hot in the rainforest-laden Maya Mountains of Belize, Central America. I was on a two-day hike into the remote and rugged main spine of the Maya Mountains proper, with some Maya healers and bushmasters out looking for sacred cacao trees (that's right, chocolate—we will talk more about this in a bit!). Anyway, we came across a large native rainforest honeybee nest and drank some of the honey. It was absolutely divine—not like honey as you would expect it, but rather like flower water. Its taste, texture and effects were exquisite—I really recall being more connected to the cosmos that day. Bees are amazing!

Ok, ok, back to the omegas…

REMINDERS ABOUT FATS

I know fats/oils get complicated. I'll try to make it easier for you. Just follow these rules to ensure healthy consumption as part of your Superfoods diet:

- get your fats/oils from Superfoods, not a bottle of oil;

- if you do use oil from a bottle use only raw, cold-pressed, unrefined oils minimally and fitting your lifestyle, and, do keep them cool and refrigerated;

- eliminate trans-fats from your diet;

- eliminate or minimize animal fats from your diet;

- plant-based saturated fats like coconut oil are beneficial, but don't overdo it;

- minimize mono/poly-unsaturated fats except for sources high in omega-3's or other rejuvenating properties;

- NO exogenous fats/oils if you have heart disease and are seeking to reverse it.

- minimal if any exogenous fats/oils if you have diabetes and are seeking to reverse it.

I want to elaborate just a bit on the first two of the aforementioned points. You should try to get your fats/oils from Superfoods, not a bottle of oil, this is because of the fact that pressed oils are highly concentrated doses of fat and Calories. Having said that, all oils are not created alike. Without writing another book here, I will tell you that provided you are rigorously adhering to the Superfoods diet, I am ok with your consuming small amounts of organic, raw, cold-pressed, unrefined oils such as coconut oil, olive oil, and sesame oil. These oils have been consumed as food and medicine in their natural and near natural, but pressed, and therefore very concentrated, forms for literally millennia by our ancestors and longest-lived elders. Similarly, I am ok with raw, cold-pressed, lignan-rich flax oil in small amounts as well. Cultures with even high intake of these specific fats exhibit significant longevity. Do not overdo it on your Superfoods diet though, you must work to minimize your intake of oils by consuming them in their natural packages and not highly concentrated forms.

A Note from Dr. Todd:

Speaking of medicinal oils, lets talk about a few:

Sesame oil is crucial to Ayurvedic medicine—it is one of the most widely used remedies of this ancient Indian healing tradition. It was, and still is, used for the gamut of ailments. Pertinent to our discussion, one of the major lignans in sesame is sesamin, which seems to ameliorate endothelial/arterial dysfunction and therefore possibly facilitates relaxation and dilation of vessels. Given the fact that endothelial dysfunction drives arterial disease, this is one important reason why sesame is an important component of the Superfoods diet.

Sesame is also a detoxifying oil used in various practices such as "pulling." Basically, pulling is a vigorous swishing of 2 tbsp. sesame oil and the pulling of it between ones teeth for approximately 15 minutes. You then spit the oil out with all of the toxins that it has pulled. In my clinical practice, this has been invaluable for a multitude of oral hygiene and other issues people have. Just as sesame oil, coconut oil has antimicrobial activity. It is another great oil for pulling and it whitens the teeth too.

On oral hygiene, do get into the habit of pulling, tongue scraping, and brushing (from the gum line to the end of the tooth) with tooth powders comprised simply of baking soda and essential oils (neem, tea tree, peppermint and birch are all great) and maybe a bit of sea salt—you can easily make your own—adding pure water to mix it all around. Also, swishing with a mild sea salt solution or pure water after eating anything is a good practice. Your teeth and gums have an ecology of their own, nurture it—optimal oral health is essential for optimal health.

In addition, do begin to learn about essential oils and health. Get yourself an essential oil diffuser and a few oils including lavender, rosemary, peppermint, cedar, sage, bee balm, clove, and grapefruit. Try giving your household or workspace a refreshing boost with some grapefruit oil in your diffuser, or a few drops of peppermint oil the next time someone has a cold or the like. Rosemary work wonders for headaches.

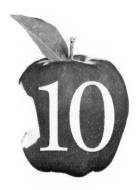

RESTORE BALANCE
TO OPTIMIZE HEALTH

By eating a diet rich in Superfoods, you will provide yourself with plenty of good carbohydrates, balanced proteins, good fats, bioavailable vitamins, minerals, trace minerals, plant pigments, enzymes, antioxidants, hormone precursors and other phytonutrients and phytochemicals, including biophotons and other essentials we have yet to uncover. Importantly, this dietary strategy and lifestyle facilitates consumption of a balanced nutritive supply to meet the demands of your physiology. This enables optimal performance, health, and wellness the way Mother Nature had intended! By eating those green leaves and rainbow veggies and fruits, along with your balanced proteins and omega-3's you're laying an excellent foundation for optimal health. Remember, since Superfoods are plant-based, nutrient-dense, calorie-sparse foods, they are health-empowering.

So eat from Dr. Todd's Superfoods Pyramid...use it as your field guide. I have my patients take it with them to the grocery store to use as a shopping guide, along with the Dirty Dozen—Clean Fifteen guide. This is your perfect foundation!

With that in mind, let's look at the top of the pyramid. In this day and age, we all fall a bit short here and there. Depleted soils, altered microbiota (both on us and in our environment), as well as toxins and stressors are all around us. Sometimes we need to help ourselves out a little…I know you know what I mean! The top of our Superfoods pyramid features those foods which help us to bridge this gap to optimal health and wellness—Functional Foods.

EAT YOUR SUPERFOODS AND SUPPLEMENT WITH FUNCTIONAL FOODS

On the Superfoods diet or any diet for that matter, I recommend responsible but intuitive supplementation as they relate to a few points of difficulty with the modern diet and lifestyle. These difficulties include: food grown in nutrient and mineral depleted soils, environmental toxins and goitrogenic antagonists (halides and others) in our water and food, and animal and animal products as part of many peoples diets—this alters gut flora (which leads to suboptimal endogenously produced nutrients) as well as unhealthful essential fatty acid ratios which drive inflammation and disease.

I first recommend regularly taking a raw, whole-foods based multivitamin to everyone: family, friends, and patients. In addition, bioavailable iodine, probiotics, digestive enzymes, vitamin D, and omega-3's in supplement form are also quite helpful. Add all that to a cupboard chock full of various herbs and spices in your Superfoods kitchen and you're on your way to functional food mastery. There are specifics below.

Don't freak out; this isn't meant to be a difficult regimen. I am not one of those types that will tell you to take a bunch of different supplements every day if you don't need them. I will, however, tell you that you do have requirements. These are necessitated by your normal physiology and your modern environment and lifestyle. Now, these requirements are ideally met through your food. If these requirements are not met through your food, they simply must be met through supplements to your food.

Just do your best. Let supplements help you out. You didn't eat green leaves yet today, don't sweat it—you can have a greens powder smoothie when you get home from your walk in the woods, your Yoga practice, or your Tai Chi in the park—throw in some chia seeds and then thank yourself for honoring you. Be good to yourself. We must supplement. This is a logical extension of balance. What we don't get here, we must get there—supplements assist us in this regard, but know what you need—know the whole how and why as well and let your body be your guide. Always remember, NO ONE, I don't care how great your doctor is, knows you better than you know yourself. Act on this and grow it… how you feel is your best guide!

A Note from Dr. Todd:

You must cultivate your way of knowing. Call it whatever you want: 6th sense, intuition, gut feeling, whatever. Textbooks speak of the 5 senses: sight, taste, touch, smell, and hearing, but cultures and wise elders the world over talk of more than this. Common everyday experience sides with the elders over the textbooks. For example, put your arm behind you, you know its there, you don't taste that it is there, nor do you hear that it is there. It is there and you know it. We have a lot of information feeds not described by the classic 5 senses. Similarly, ever meet someone who you really like and know it right off the bat? Or conversely, been creeped out by some situation, but can't explain why, then have it confirmed later? That's your intuition talking to you. Truly, this sense, your gut, is like a second brain—honor it as such! Further, the gut is home to a vibrant ecosystem of microbes that do a heck of a lot more than help digest your food. We will talk more about this in a bit.

So, while the majority of our requirements are abundant in our Superfoods diet and lifestyle, there are some areas where we need extra assurance that our requirements are being met.

- Our nutritional requirements are complicated. Science has uncovered a great deal of truth with regard to our physiologies and biochemistry. However, there is still a majority of truth out there that has yet to be elucidated. In meeting our optimal nutritional requirements, I advocate for following the Superfoods diet and lifestyle of our longest-lived elders and our ancestors for the wisdom of our cultures speaks volumes through them. I don't have to know the ins and outs of everything, because time has tested them.

- You don't have to Calorie count or vitamin and mineral count on a Superfoods diet. It is not Calorie restrictive—only in that it excludes certain foods that serve no purpose in your body and it limits unnatural concentrations of nutrients such as fats and sugars. You can eat as many Superfoods as your body tells you that you need. Dial in to your cravings—oftentimes your body will tell you when and what it needs to eat. Sometimes your body will direct you to grazing, so eat a bit here and there—as long as it is Superfoods you are eating. Trust yourself.

- The diversity of Superfoods, as the pyramid illustrates, will facilitate adequate nutrient intake for optimal health. Further, the nutrient intake is in its ideal plant-based form. This, for example, makes the nutrients we require more bioavailable—minerals are taken from the soil into the plant where they are chelated, making them more useful to you. Remember, the soil becomes us via the plants.

- The Superfoods diet places our physiologies where they are best suited to function and thereby enables the maintenance of homeostasis more optimally. It meets our biochemistry where it functions best.

A Note from Dr. Todd:

Back to the balance thing... We need our feeding states to be interspersed with those of fasting. We need our periods of activity to be interspersed with inactivity, of socialization with solitude and introspection, and our mentation with its purposeful antithesis—keep that in mind. I have noticed that with monotony comes translocation. People are translocated to the past and depressed... you know these are the could have, should have types. Or people are translocated to the future and anxious... these are the what if this, what if that types. Ground yourself in the present, for this is the only moment that is life. This infinite experience is all yours all now. As the elders teach, presence in the present will provide for your future. Meditation, Yoga, Tai Chi, and walks in the woods (nature in general) help with this.

There are all these fad diets and lots of conflicting information out there. Let how you feel guide your practices—learn from your Superfoods facilitated radiance.

Here are my basic starting point recommendations for dietary supplementation. I make these recommendations to every new patient at my practice. Rarely do they stay the same; rather, they are continually fine-tuned with my guidance and based on how that particular patient is feeling, but it is a starting point for you. I tell my patients they need to intuit their needs—after all, no one knows your body better than you! For example, I take my various supplements when I feel that I need them—usually 2-6 times a week in the morning—sometimes none though—I give myself a break. Sometimes I take additional items in the afternoon. Here and there I will take a sublingual B12 supplement for a few weeks, sometimes I will up my D, or my iodine. I notice that in times of illness and/or stressors, I need more—so might you. Once you have followed your Superfoods diet and given yourself time to tune in, I suggest you move things around to suit your particular needs on that day.

Further, I find the whole thrice or even twice-daily dosing requirements written on the packaging of many supplements to be challenging for most, and, quite frankly, overdone—even ludicrous at times. I mean seriously, come on now… as my elders would say, "you won't shrivel up and blow away if you don't eat today"—by extension we are likely quite good without 24-7 coverage of a multivitamin. I know the water-soluble vitamins have a half-life of under 24 hours—in other words, they are peed out quickly—but who cares? You are eating often enough and you store vitamins and minerals. Therefore, your body will be just fine if you accidentally miss your twice-daily multivitamin.

WHAT TO TAKE

To begin, try:

- A good Multivitamin with B12 (derived from whole foods, raw is best) ideally twice a day.

Avoid synthetic vitamins. They are obviously not natural and I am not surprised that studies have shown synthetic vitamins may well increase the risk of cancer. In particular, synthetic beta-carotene, and vitamin E—I highlight these two since there is extant data on them, other synthetics will likely be proven similarly detrimental to our health in the future. Stick to whole foods and whole foods supplements—just as Mother Nature intends!

- Occasional B12 sublingually or even intramuscularly; you might want to have your B12 level checked periodically,

- Bioavailable Iodine 3 mg or so a day,

- A good Probiotic on an empty stomach just prior to going to bed, and,

- Vitamin D 5000 IU daily (once levels optimized and checking periodically).

We know that if we spent more time naked in the sunshine as our ancestors have done then we would meet our requirements for D—given modern day realities, we choose to balance this requirement with supplementation.

- Plant-based omega-3's (flax, chia and/or walnuts) 3.5 grams of omega-3's daily as a minimum,

- Algae-based DHA 150 mg daily, and,

- Plant-based digestive enzymes with meals, in particular larger meals and evening meals when needed.

Now let's get into the specifics of two essential supplements. I recommend them for a reason!

VITAMIN B12

Vitamin B12 is the main reason I recommend a daily whole foods multivitamin. I aim for a minimum of 100 mcg of B12 daily in the multivitamin. The absorption mechanics for vitamin B12 are complex and involve uptake in your small intestine when bound to a special protein. Vitamin B12 is an extremely large and complicated molecule; because of this we absorb only a small amount of this crucial nutrient. It is essential to our health functioning in diverse fashion for neurological health, immune system health, energy and even sleep.

Vitamin B12 is kind of similar to Nitrogen in the sense that it is made available to plants and people by microbes found in the soil and on plants and people. Basically, animals (us included) eat these microbes as we take in our food; they then transiently make their homes in our small intestines, where B12 is absorbed, and while there they give us a bit of this crucial nutrient for absorption.

The modern-day human doesn't eat their daily dose of these microbes, whereas the other modern-day animals continue to do so. There are multiple reasons for this including the fact that the odd practice of obsessively cleaning vegetables and even peeling off their skin prior to eating is only done by humans.

To contrast this, I grew up eating dirty veggies (good dirt—soil) from field and forest just as my ancestors have done and just as my children do now. They are health empowering with a bit of good old Mother Earth as nature intends. No, no, we do not eat mud pies, nor are our veggies covered in soil, but they are not obsessively over-cleaned either, they are eaten right off of the plants. Of course, we give the root veggies a rinse, and we wash our produce from the grocery store and other markets, but the point is we need a bit of good dirt! Further, microbes are scarce on plants we eat now because of the preponderance of pesticides, herbicides, fungicides and other chemicals unfortunately used in modern-agriculture.

There is no question our ancestors ate more good dirt, microbes and even insects (which have significant concentrations of vitamin B12) with their Superfoods—much more so than we do in the modern-day. This is a major way they got their B12. Of note, they also ate a lot of mushrooms. Mushrooms are crucial in the Superfoods diet for a multitude of reasons including the fact that they have considerable amounts of B12.

So, basically, in our modern-day Superfoods diet, there are not enough of these good microbes on our plant-based foods to ensure regular inoculation of our small bowel. In the modern-day, most people get their B12 from animal products; the animals get B12 from microbes they eat with their food. However, recent studies show that almost half of the United States population is B12 deficient, yet they consume plenty of animal products on SAD. Why?

B12 (or cobalamin) requires cobalt. The microbes complex cobalt in the B12 molecule. Our soils are becoming more and more depleted. Less cobalt, less cobalamin for all animals, us included. I don't care whether you eat animal products or not, either way you likely need B12 supplementation.

A Note from Dr. Todd:

The human large and small intestine harbor a considerable microflora ecosystem that we are reliant on for health. Maintaining a plant-based Superfoods diet results in a significant shift in the inhabitants of this flora (while total cell numbers remain the same) for the better in terms of optimal health. We now know that at least two groups of microorganisms which inhabit the small intestine, *Pseudomonas* sp., and *Klebsiella* sp., synthesize significant amounts of B12. Our bowel flora shifts in relation to a number of factors—it is in delicate balance. In nature, animals (for example, rabbits) will oftentimes resort to eating their own, or others, feces to regain some B12 that has gone unabsorbed. If you have ever wondered why your dog licks their friend's behind, this is likely a part of their instinctive drive to replenish B12.

IODINE

Seaweeds are amazing Superfoods—be sure to chow down on this oceanic goodness often. You can meet your iodine requirements through them if you'd like. In my view, there is unfounded trepidation with regard to iodine supplementation. Many regularly ingest whopping amounts of iodine, even in the range of hundreds of milligrams (mg) daily without noticeable adverse effects. In my experience, what your body does not need, it will eliminate. Further, the average SAD has on the order of micrograms (mcg) of iodine daily whereas the average Japanese diet has on the order of mg daily—thousands of times more! Recall the life expectancy comparison I drew earlier in the book, and note their more plant-based diet AND lack of a major preponderance of thyroid disorders relative to the United States—a root of concern for iodine supplementation. Bottom line: our ancestors ate a good amount of iodine, and so should you. They ate it in the form of mineral salts, root veggies and seaweed for the most part—these all concentrate iodine. You can get it that way or take a bioavailable iodine supplement.

STRESS, INFLAMMATION AND OXIDATIVE STRESSORS: A FEW KEY FUNCTIONAL FOODS

Ok, so we have supplemented. What's next? While I realize a comprehensive listing of functional foods, herbs, and spices is virtually impossible (and also out of the scope of this book), I would like to share a few of my favorites with you. These items are important for dealing with the negative effects of stress, inflammation, and oxidative stressors (discussed when we learned about plant pigments).

- **Maitake**. *Hen-of-the-Woods*, or *Ram's Head*—you all might be more familiar with its widely known Japanese name, *Maitake*, which means "dancing mushroom." This name stems from the fact that when people found them they were overjoyed and so driven to dancing a bit in the woods. The scientific name is *Grifola frondosa*, and it is a choice edible species. It is a polypore mushroom, meaning it drops spores from holes underneath rather than gills. It is easy to identify as it looks like a ruffled hen in the woods (as the name would suggest). Notably, there aren't any poisonous species that look quite like it. Recently, science has begun to recognize the healing properties of these magic mushrooms so spoken of by our ancestors. An explosion of research spearheaded in Japan has corroborated the powerful, supportive medicinal effects of mushrooms on one's immune system, and on cancer in particular. They also help out with sugar regulation. Maitake mushrooms contain certain types of polysaccharides (recall that's a chain of sugar molecules), called beta-glucans. Beta-glucans are found in several different types of mushrooms and are believed to stimulate the immune system and activate cells and proteins that attack cancer, including natural killer cells, macrophages and T-cells—all that and they are quite delicious! Definitely worth dancing in the woods for all of that!

- **Maca.** Maca, or *Lepidium peruvianum* Chacon is a Superfood grown in the high Andes (mainly Peru and Bolivia). It grows as a root that tastes a little like butterscotch, and is packed with vitamins, minerals, proteins, complex alkaloids and other beneficial phytochemicals. Maca is highly nutritious, being comprised in majority of balanced carbohydrates combined with roughly 10-15% protein and about 2% or so fat (of which EFA's are a significant component). It is also a rich source of plant sterols. From a mineral standpoint, maca exceeds both potatoes and carrots in value, and is a source of iron, magnesium, calcium, potassium, and iodine. Maca is often consumed in its powdered root form.

As a result of this extensive nutritional profile and its phytochemical constituents, maca enhances mental clarity, physical strength, and stamina. On a physical level, maca has been used by indigenous cultures (in particular the Inca) for physical stamina, such as before athletic events, battle, and bedroom activities! It increases not only one's desire for physical activity, but the ability to accomplish it as well. Maca is an excellent adaptogen—meaning it does for your body what you need done; helping to balance the body's systems under physical and emotional stress is one of its key characteristics. This, in turn, has a positive effect on healthful awareness, memory, clarity, stamina, thyroid function, hormonal balance, and physical energy. As maca helps support endocrine function, it is perhaps an excellent way to offset the disruptive effects of environmental toxin exposure. I know quite a few people who rely on maca to get them through difficult days—my sister calls it "Mother's Little Helper", and it is a lifesaver for menopause. It is, without a doubt, an amazing complement to your Superfoods program.

A Peruvian shaman once said to me "A day without maca is a day without sunshine." I can tell you that I have many patients who would agree! Several of my favorite maca testimonials include:

- "I can now find my keys whenever I need them!",

- "It has given me my sex life back!" (My friends and I have a running joke that maca is responsible for all of our families! Yeah, it is that good!), and

- "I won my first 5K!"

- "It has rekindled my marriage!"

A Note from Dr. Todd:

Maca is amazing, but you ever been "Sang-in" in the mountains? American Ginseng is another miraculous plant. Most people are surprised to learn that we have been exporting our native Appalachian ginseng to China for hundreds of years! *Panax quinquefolius* is remarkable—talk about strength, stamina and mental clarity! This is definitely another to add to your Superfoods armamentarium!

- **Cat's Claw.** Cat's Claw, or *Uncaria tomentosa*, is named for the cat's claw-like spines located on the underside of the leaves of this woody vine. It is native to much of the neotropics where it is used widely as a sacred medicinal plant and in treatment of the gamut of ailments. Scientifically, cat's claw has been shown to be immunomodulatory in nature. Basically, it is an inhibitor of certain immune system components which stimulate TNF alpha, an inflammatory mediator in our bodies, and which is responsible for inflammation, and, in part, the aforementioned diseases of civilization. TNF alpha is also involved with autoimmune conditions such as inflammatory bowel disease, psoriasis, and certain types of arthritis. In my clinical practice, cat's claw has been tremendously effective in relief from these and other conditions. In addition, cat's claw has antioxidant properties and is an excellent bowel cleanser which helps to reset proper flora balance in the intestines. As a result, cat's claw enhances the normal physiologic functioning, lymphatic drainage, and detoxification of the body.

In the World Health Organization-sponsored First International Conference on this species, it was pointed out that no other rainforest plant has ever prompted such worldwide attention since quinine was discovered in the bark of a Peruvian tree in the 17th century. Indigenous peoples worldwide such as the Maya cultures of the Central American rainforests and the Ashaninkas, Huitoto, Bora, Yahua, Campas and Amueshas of Amazonia have been using this plant for its diverse healing properties and as directed by their shamans and healers for many generations. Per the Maya healers I work with in Belize, it is one of the three most sought after plants (Because I know you're curious, the other two are "man stick", a phallic looking plant with the biologic function of, well, you know. The other is a *Dioscorea* sp. It's a type of wild yam which is used in birth control).

Do not use cat's claw if you are pregnant, or if there is any possibility you are pregnant, or if you are trying to get pregnant. It is used traditionally in a number of applications including in birth control and as an abortifactant.

HERBS AND SPICES: SEASON YOUR FOOD AND SPICE UP YOUR PALATE

Seasoning our food not only makes it taste wonderful, but also has an impact on our well being! Many of the widely used herbs and spices have therapeutic properties. With regard to these seasonings, diversity is key. Use all sorts of different herbs and spices, not just mineral sea salt and black pepper. Herbs and Spices are Superfoods Superstars and you need plenty of them. Be adventurous! And don't be afraid to ask questions of your friends, your grocer, your international restaurant favorites—and don't forget the gold standard: your library or internet. We have wonderful ethnic markets in the Cleveland area. If you have the same near you, go and explore and ask questions.

When speaking of these herbs, please don't take capsules or pills—eat the real thing. No garlic or turmeric capsules—cook with garlic. Cook with turmeric. The health benefits of the whole plant, as we discussed earlier, far outweigh the benefits of any capsule. Having said that, if you need to supplement, by all means please do…that is better than nothing.

Speaking of **turmeric**, or the root-stem of *Curcuma longa,* this spice has been used in India for millennia, and contains potent healing properties. It is an amazing health rejuvenating, anti-inflammatory blessing of a plant. One active component, curcumin, is found to be most effective when combined with black pepper—two key ingredients in many delicious curry recipes. See that, once again the ancestors and elders are right! I recommend adding this combination of spices to a regular rotation in your kitchen—have a delicious curry or turmeric dish at least two to three times weekly. There are great recipes available all over the place…be creative!

A Note from Dr. Todd:

Curry is a general term used to describe a diverse mix of spices used as food and medicine, originally throughout Asia and now worldwide. The major spices found in curries are turmeric, cumin, black pepper, and coriander—there are lots of others. I have eaten curries with over 100 spices blended. Talk about divinity of the palate!

I am thinking of this time when I was on a bus in Kerala, India. I had this wicked head cold that had been lingering for about 4 or 5 days then, as I was headed across the Western Ghats Mountains from Coimbatore to Thiruvananthapuram (capital of Kerala). Through the window passed startlingly beautiful country punctuated with rolling tea plantations, sandalwood forests, and wild elephants!

I arrived in sought-after Munnar, in all its majestic splendor, and all I wanted to do was sleep. I got off the bus to the greetings of a yogi friend. He looked at me, and a millisecond later, he said, smiling, "Come, you are not well."

After showing me to my accommodations, he brought me a warm beverage consisting of loads of turmeric, ginger, black pepper, and long pepper (another type of pepper similar to black pepper, only much hotter) among other things. I drank it down. It was delicious… then I was out. I had some very powerful dreams that night. After about 10 hours of sleep, I woke feeling wonderful. Not a trace of the cold. It was completely gone.

Ginger is the rhizome (stem-root) of *Zingiber officinale*. It is consumed in foods, as a plant medicine, and as a spice. It is related to turmeric, galangal and cardamom. As a versatile root spice, it works well in both sweet and savory preparation, and is known for its gastrointestinal benefits and anti-inflammatory properties. In fact, studies have linked ginger to a reduction in colorectal cancer incidence.

Bitter greens and herbs that we have used to season our food have been supporting our health for millennia. Some contemporary, locally grown favorites of mine include: garlic, onion, chives, basil, oregano, rosemary, thyme, marjoram, tarragon, dill, cilantro, parsley and sage. These have been flavoring our food AND improving our health for generations. A great many age-old seasonings contain these "revolutionary" healing plants and their properties, so it is essential to eat a wide range of flavors. A benefit to this is that your palate will never get bored!

Culinary herbs such as these are nearly foolproof to grow and do not take much space to cultivate, so consider an herb patch in your yard or a window herb garden. Local herbs are normally in abundance at your farmer's market, too, and can be dried and stored if purchased in large quantities.

Further, no household should be without the medicinal herb garden compliment to the aforementioned culinary herbs. Try growing cayenne peppers, yarrow, bee balm, *Echinacea* sp., peppermint and spearmint (note these last two will take over, so plant them in their own space), and lemon balm. These are all easy to grow and are quite rewarding. A few others you might want to try involve a bit of cultivation in the woods—you can try to seed a ramp patch, or plant some ginseng and some goldenseal. While there are many, many more, that's a start. You're on your way in Appalachian root doctoring!

A Note from Dr. Todd:

I grew up going outside to chew on an echinacea root at first sign of a cold. It really is a miraculous plant teacher (If that didn't work there was always the echinacea-goldenseal brew ever warming on our wood-burning stove. And, if there was present a bit of a sore throat of course cherry bark and slippery elm would do the trick). There are all kinds of echinacea, as well as other roots, shoots, leaves and the like and all kinds of ways to prepare them. The important first step is to grow some. Respect these beings, and then begin to learn of the different types.

CHOCOLATE AND TEA: LIFE'S SIMPLE PLEASURES

Cacao. Yes, chocolate! Chocolate is made from the fermented, dried seeds of a tree which grows in the rainforest (*Theobroma cacao* of the family Malvaceae). Cacao is known to be one of the highest dietary sources of magnesium and contains an impressively high iron content. Cacao has more antioxidant flavonoids than most green teas!

Chocolate also:

- supports healthful circulation and blood pressure, since it is rich in theobromine and magnesium, which are vasodilators;

- is a stimulant, theobromine;

- contains tryptophan which supports serotonin, a neurotransmitter that acts in our brain similarly to an anti-depressant;

- contains phenylethylamine, a feel-good neurotransmitter which promotes feelings of love;

- contains anandamide, which facilitates feelings of wellbeing, relaxation and bliss; and

- contains sulfur, calcium, zinc, iron, copper, folic acid, vitamins A, E, K and potassium.

Whew, all that psychoactivity induced vasodilation, bliss, and love—that's a party! And, that is exactly what the ancient Maya believed. They revered chocolate as a food of the gods. All of this supports healthful blood pressure, healthful aging and mood, and a healthful immune system response. It also increases alertness and awareness.

The closer to the raw, dark form of cacao you can get, the more nutrients and better effects you will have. Eating highly processed chocolate bars will not provide all of the above benefits (besides, they are loaded with sugar). Go with the raw or dark chocolates. There is a chocolatier in all of us! Explore your region and see who's doing great things with dark chocolate. Then eat some!

Matcha Green Tea. Along with eating chocolate, enjoy a daily cup of green tea. My recommendation is matcha green tea. Matcha is green tea leaves in powdered form. It is uniquely Japanese and is the highest quality tea available in Japan, where it is a known anti-cancer agent.

- Matcha, or rubbed tea, was first used by Buddhist monks for religious rituals in the 12th century. This ceremonial green tea comes from the careful harvesting methods of the finest tea leaves grown in Uji, Japan. It is one of a variety of green teas made from young Gyokuro (or Jade Dew), *Camellia sinensis,* leaves. One glass of matcha is the equivalent of many more cups of infused green tea in terms of its nutritional value and antioxidant content.

- Matcha is full of cancer fighting antioxidants. We discussed these in our rainbow veggies and fruits chapter, so you already know that not all antioxidants are the same. The antioxidants in matcha are in the family called catechins (which are found predominantly in green tea). Of that family, a principle catechin in green tea is epigallocatechin gallate, or EGCG, which contains strong antioxidant and cancer fighting properties. Sixty percent of the antioxidants in matcha are EGCGs.

I am often asked about drinking coffee vs. consuming green tea. Understandably, some prefer to avoid caffeine. Here's what I tell them: matcha provides minerals, vitamins (A, various B vitamins, C, E, and K), and, like all green teas, does contain a small amount of caffeine, but also contains L-theanine, an amino acid known to promote healthful mood and feelings of well being. L-theanine increases the alpha wave activities in the brain, creating a feeling of relaxation and ease. L-theanine is associated with increased ability to focus, but does not create nervousness or agitation. This is due to the whole package delivery of the phytonutrients as well as the consumption method of the green tea which helps to balance the caffeine and ensure a more balanced absorption through digestion. This means you have no "jittery" feelings often associated with coffee and suffer no "drop off" effect as it leaves your system. Matcha is also alkaline as compared to acidic (like coffee) and therefore does not have the negative effect of coffee on the stomach and gastrointestinal system. As if that weren't enough, matcha also contains chlorophyll which is an anti-inflammatory, an antioxidant, and also good for detoxification and purification.

It is a great way to switch out coffee. My patients love it! I have not yet encountered one single person with coffee-caffeine sensitivity that is unable to drink matcha and feel great. All that and it facilitates your daily meditative space—remember—drink your tea slowly, reverently and in the present.

LAST THOUGHTS: SUPER YOU IN ALL ASPECTS

Hair analyses are excellent clinical tools for assessing minerals and even preliminarily screening for toxic heavy metals. One can also determine certain metabolic specifics from mineral profiles as well. I have all of my patients get one annually. We track their progress through them and this strategy works out quite well. A good resource for hair analyses is Trace Elements, Inc. If there is evidence of toxic heavy metals in a hair analysis, I further recommend that they have a more rigorous assessment of heavy metal burden through a Urine Toxic Metals provocative assessment analyzed by Doctors Data. Remember, as unfortunate as it is, in this day and age, it is impossible to exist in a toxic free environment. However, it is not impossible to approach a toxic free you. This requires some effort: Superfoods diet and lifestyle including regular cleansing. I recommend to all of my patients that they cleanse twice a year. Once in the spring, and once in the fall—view these as internal house keeping, just as one must spring clean prior to the fresh summer air and put away fall clutter moving into the winter months.

In addition to your Superfoods Diet and Lifestyle already discussed, do consider:

- Cleansing twice annually at a minimum (spring and fall)

    - At my practice, I regularly use juice and water fasting; Standard Process 21 Day Purification Program, Dairy Free (with some additions of my own); Master Cleanse (with some additions/ adjustments of my own); and Apple Cleansing for Liver/Gallbladder flushing and other cleansing with good results.

- Colon Hydrotherapy

- Biomeridian Assessment

- Electromagnetic and energetic body work

- Homeopathy

- Chlorella and algae

- Zeolites

- Chelation

- Megavitamin repletion therapy for vitamin D and B12

- Bioidentical Hormones Balancing (plant-based)

- Sauna (infrared has deepest penetration)—be sure to rinse off afterward to clean toxins off your body

- Massage and lymphatic drainage

- Acupuncture

I know you will find your journey and residence in the Superfoods lifestyle rewarding as you will experience a renewed, healthy, vital existence! I look forward to sharing that journey with you as you Eat Yourself Super using the guidelines throughout this publication. I'd love to hear from you regarding your voyage! Be well.

ABOUT THE AUTHOR

Todd J. Pesek, M.D. is a holistic physician and published scholar who specializes in disease prevention and reversal toward longevity and vital living.

He is in private practice in northeastern, Ohio, and is co-founder of group medical practice *Great Lakes Health Institute* of Lyndhurst, Ohio, which focuses on preventive, integrative, holistic healthcare. Dr. Pesek is also a tenured Health Sciences Professor at *Cleveland State University*, Cleveland, Ohio, where he teaches, researches and serves in multiple capacities, including as founding Director for the *Center for Healing Across Cultures*. In addition, he is founder of leading organic Superfoods and herbals companies *Dr. Todd's Superfoods* and *Earth Healers*.

Dr. Todd was raised in the mountains of Appalachia in rural Pennsylvania and embraced his calling of holistic health and wellness from an early age. His passion and purpose began in the woods; gathering comfort and learning truth from his elders and the Earth. These adventures blossomed into extensive study and collaboration with traditional healers and holistic health practitioners in places as far away as India, Peru and Belize. His goal is to shed light on holistic health and wellness through timeless healing traditions that have long helped us maintain personal health and wellness, and can help us stay healthy and filled with vitality today. His work illustrates how we all can achieve wellness through hydration, Superfoods nutrition, alkalinization, and detoxification, and that an immersion into nature, the healing plants and traditional practices of the world allow this true health.

Dr. Todd received his medical doctorate from The Ohio State University College of Medicine and the Cleveland Clinic in Cleveland, Ohio, and completed his training in Medicine at Case Western Reserve University School of Medicine, St. Vincent Charity Hospital, Cleveland, Ohio.

To read more about Dr. Todd, visit his blog at: www.healingspaceblog.com.

NOTES

1. T.C. Campbell and T.M. Campbell II, *The China Study*, BenBella Books, 2005

2. C.B. Esselstyn Jr., "Updating a 12 -Year Experience With Arrest and Reversal Therapy for Coronary Heart Disease (An Overdue Requiem for Palliative Cardiology)." *The Am J of Cardiology.* 1999; 84:339-341

3. C.B. Esselstyn Jr., "Resolving the Coronary Artery Disease Epidemic through Plant-Based Nutrition." *Preventive Cardiology.* 2001; 4:171-177

4. D. Ornish, L.W. Scherwitz, J.H., Billings et al. "Intensive Lifestyle Changes for Reversal of Coronary Heart Disease." *JAMA.* 1998; 280:2001-2007

5. W.C. Willett, "Balancing life-style and genomics research for disease prevention." *Science.* 2002; 296:695-698

6. C. Gorman, A. Park, K. Dell. "Health: The Fires Within" *Time Magazine.* 2004; 163(8):7-12

7. C.B. Esselstyn Jr., *Prevent and Reverse Heart Disease,* Penguin Group, 2007

8. D. Ornish, *Dr. Dean Ornish's Program for Reversing Heart Disease: The Only System Scientifically Proven to Reverse Heart Disease Without Drugs or Surgery,* Ballantine Books, 1996

9. N. Barnard, *Dr. Neal Barnard's Program for Reversing Diabetes,* Rodale, 2007

10. R. Mano, A. Ishida, Y. Ohya, et al. "Dietary intervention with Okinawan vegetables increased circulating endothelial progenitor cells in healthy young women." *Atherosclerosis.* 2009; 204(2):544-8

11. S.R. Smith, "A Look at the Low-Carbohydrate Diet." *N Engl J Med.* 2009; 361:2286-2288

12. American Diabetes Association. Diabetes Basics. Accessed: October 5, 2011 at http://www.diabetes.org/diabetes-basics/type-2/

13. P. Melpomeni, J. Uribarri, H. Vlassara, "Glucose, Advanced Glycation End Products, and Diabetes Complications: What Is New and What Works." *Clinical Diabetes.* 2003; 21(4):186-187

14. K.R. Smith, C.F. Corvalan, T. Kjellstrom. "How much global ill health is attributable to environmental factors?" *Epidemiology.* 1999; 10:573-84

15. WHO. Environmental burden of disease: country profiles Geneva. WHO. 2007. www.who.int/quantifying_ehimpacts/countryprofiles/en/index.html

16. A.H. Mokdad, J.S. Marks, D.F. Stroup et al. Actual causes of death in the U.S., 2000. *JAMA.* 2005; 293(3):293-4.

17. N. Kilpatrick, H. Frumkin, J. Trowbridge et al. The environmental history in pediatric practice: a study of pediatricians' attitudes, beliefs, and practices. *Environ Health Perspect.* 2002; 110(8):823-7

18. A. Pruss-Ustun, C. Corvalan. Preventing disease through healthy environments. Towards an estimate of the environmental burden of disease. Geneva, Switzerlands: WHO, 2006

19. Environmental Working Group. *Body Burdon—The pollution in newborns,* 2005. Retrieved 05/22/2010 from: http://www.ewg.org/reports/bodyburden2/execsumm.php

20. Experimental Man. Main Page, 2011. Retrieved 10/08/2011 from: http://www.experimentalman.com/

21. R. Deitsch and S. Lonky, *Invisible Killers: The truth about environmental genocide.* Invisible Killer Enterprises, 2007

22. B. Lipton, *The Biology of Belief.* Hay House, 2005

23. D. Ornish, M.J. Magbanua, G. Weidner et al. "Changes in prostate gene expression in men undergoing an intensive nutrition and lifestyle intervention." *Proc Natl Acad Sci.* 2008; 105(24):8369-74

24. D. Ornish, J. Lin, J. Daubenmier, et al. "Increased telomerase activity and comprehensive lifestyle changes: a pilot study." *Lancet Oncol.* 2008;9:1048-1057

25. T. Pesek, R. Reminick, M. Nair, "Secrets of Long Life: Cross-Cultural Explorations in Sustainably Enhancing Vitality and Promoting Longevity Via Elders' Practice Wisdom." *Explore.* 2010; 6(6):352-358

26. Campbell and Campbell. Pg 229.

APPENDIX

SUPERFOODS RECIPES
A Note from the Superfoods Kitchen:

I compiled the following recipes with YOU in mind, a person working to make small, albeit important, changes in your diet and lifestyle, and perhaps also in the diet and lifestyle of your family. I asked my wife, Leah to assist me in this regard as the Superfoods journey is not a road easily taken alone in the family setting and her experience and wisdom as a long-time Superfoods mom and wife can add invaluably to the practicality and feasibility of your Superfoods endeavors.

While I want to bring our Superfoods kitchen into your home—I want to do so as healthfully, easily and deliciously as possible. The goal here is to demonstrate some healthy alternatives to SAD staples—to ease your transition. I have aimed to steer clear of overwhelming you by gathering recipes that contain foods which are first and foremost Superfoods, and are furthermore realistic, accessible, obtainable, and easy to prepare—they are all family friendly. They are also great shared romantically with a loved one, or even eaten alone—they are quite versatile. They are a beginning—a realistic starting point for your journey. You have grown accustomed to eating a particular way and now you are ready to change, these will help to facilitate this change, but will require constant evolution to fit your unique needs.

The recipes are organized roughly (as there is a lot of overlap in Superfoods) according to Dr. Todd's Superfoods Pyramid (see Appendix) and run the gamut of meal type: from smoothie, to juice, to snack, to side dish, entrée choice, and even dessert. Assume the meals are designed to feed four people, unless otherwise noted.

When you see "olive oil", "sesame oil", or "coconut oil", I am referring ONLY to organic, cold-pressed, extra virgin oils, and when you see "sea salt", I am referring to mineral sea salt such as Celtic Light Grey Sea Salt or Real Salt. Note, olive oil, sesame oil, and coconut oil are highly concentrated fat (and associated Calories) and while they are healthier fats with even healthful or medicinal properties, they are not good for you in excess. Remember, for the most part, excess is anything more than that which can be taken in via consuming food in its natural form. Therefore, use these oils sparingly (but fitting the rest of your diet and lifestyle). Also, keep in mind that the best oil to cook with is coconut oil (followed by olive and sesame).

Similarly, salt in excess is not good; but pure, mineral sea salt such as the aforementioned contains many trace minerals which are vital to good health. So, when you see "salt to taste" in a recipe, don't hold back—just don't overdo it!

As always, use as many local, organic foods as possible. You will need to get a mortar and pestle (no one should be without!) to crush and grind garlic, and other fresh and dried herbs and spices. And, do remember to ALWAYS refer to your Soaking and Sprouting Chart (see Appendix) whenever you see seeds, nuts and legumes. Unless otherwise noted, sprouting and soaking is implicit in all following recipes.

Learn to steam sauté to reduce your oils and to keep your food raw or as raw as possible—you can eat warm food without devitalizing it. And, do NOT use aluminum, non-stick skillets or cooking sprays as they are toxic. Cook or warm food only in glass, stainless steel or cast iron. And, forget about microwaving anything. If you have one, get rid of it—fast!

Please remember that cooking or more importantly preparing Superfoods in the RAW is easy and fun once you get into the swing of things! This will get you started. It is not an exact science; feel free to add a little more of this or that, or get creative and add something not even listed in the recipes. This is how we do it in our house; it is what Leah's grandmother calls "cooking pizzazza." Do get a feel for your food and prepare it with LOVE.

I strive to show you that a plant-based lifestyle is not out of your reach—and you and your children will adore it, as do we. Remember, love people—feed them Superfoods! Before you know it, your dinner parties will fill as fast as ours! Bon Appétit!

A few more points to consider:

- Remember, when combating fat and sugar toxicities, fat or sugar outside of their natural plant-based forms must be minimized if not eliminated.

  - If you have heart disease and are seeking to reverse it, you cannot have any fat. None! Similarly, if you have diabetes, you must avoid sugar and high GI foods, you must also minimize fat.

- If you must use a sweetener use grade B maple syrup, fresh squeezed orange juice, green coconut water, raw coconut nectar, stevia, or raw honey as these are relatively low GI sweeteners with wide applicability and are quite yummy! Do NOT use artificial sweeteners as they are toxic.

  - While Agave Nectar is a low GI sweetener this is misleading. It is low GI because it contains unnaturally high concentrations of fructose relative to glucose and therefore largely bypasses a key regulatory checkpoint in sugar metabolism. In essence, on consuming, it is metabolized whether we need it or not—this is why it is low GI, because it doesn't hang around in the blood, it is channel stuffed elsewhere (and this causes additional problems). This is also why high fructose corn syrup is bad for you.

- **Eat RAW Superfoods as much as you can**. In essence, a diversity of raw Superfoods are the cornerstone to your health.

  - Get your Superfoods kitchen set up for this—it is much easier that way.

    » Buy your Superfoods in bulk—lots!

    » Get a good blender or VitaMix

    » Get a good juicer or Champion Juicer

    » Get a good dehydrator or Excalibur (A low temp oven is an acceptable temporary fix.)

    » Get organic cheese cloth and a bunch of sprout jars

    » Get a mortar and pestle

» Get a good raw foods book. <u>Raw: The Uncook Book</u> by Juliano is an excellent choice.

» Get a good fermented foods book. <u>Wild Fermentation: The Flavor, Nutrition, and Craft of Live-Culture Foods</u> by Sandor Ellix Katz is one such reference.

» Shopping Staples (local, organic first):
  + Lots of greens
  + Lots of rainbow veggies
  + Lots of rainbow fruits
  + Lots of fresh and dried herbs and spices
  + Bulk dried seeds, nuts and legumes
  + Quinoa
  + Chia, flax and walnuts
  + Lemons
  + Wild and brown rice
  + Sprouted grain bread and wraps
  + Fresh gourmet mushrooms
  + Seaweed (wakame, kelp, dulse, nori)
  + Raw Cacao Nibs (Chocolate)
  + Matcha Green Tea
  + Maca
  + Ohsawa Nama Shoyu (good soy sauce)
  + Olive oil (keep refrigerated)
  + Sesame oil (keep refrigerated)
  + Sesame seeds
  + Tahini (keep refrigerated)
  + Coconut oil (best oil for cooking)
  + Grade B Maple Syrup
  + Bragg Raw Apple Cider Vinegar
  + Mineral sea salt such as Celtic Light Grey Sea Salt or Real Salt
  + Black pepper
  + Turmeric
  + Curry powders

+ Ginger
+ Cinnamon

FIRST AND FOREMOST! MAKE THESE:

SUPERBROTH

For every 2 gallons of pure water add:

1 medium red onion

1 medium white onion

2 medium carrots

8 celery stalks

8 cloves garlic

1 medium daikon radish (root and tops), optional but ideal

1 small butternut or other winter squash (in winter) *or*

1 medium zucchini and 1 medium yellow squash (in summer)

1 Spanish black radish, optional but ideal

1 medium red or golden beet (root and tops)

1 medium turnip (root and tops)

1 bunch kale (your choice)

1 bunch parsley

1 bunch cilantro

½ bunch rainbow chard

½ bunch mustard greens

½ cup dried seaweed (wakame, kelp, dulse, or nori) (1 cup if fresh)

½ small red cabbage

½ small green cabbage

1 lemon (cut in half)

1 thumb sized piece of ginger minced

2 tsp. turmeric

1 cup dried maitake or shiitake mushrooms (two cups if fresh)

1 tbsp. sea salt

1 tsp. black pepper

2 cayenne peppers

Steps: Chop all ingredients except for cayenne pepper and garlic (add these whole) along with all other ingredients at once and place on a low simmer for approximately 1 hour. Depending on exact ingredients and seasonality, it may take a bit longer. Once done, allow to cool on stove for few hours then strain (you can eat the cooked vegetables, they are great dehydrated, you can also dehydrate your juiced veggie pulp—these are both awesome sources of dietary fiber). Store the broth in a large glass container that is well sealed in your fridge. Gallon jugs work well. You can warm gently and drink 2-4 cups a day. Also, this serves as a great base, and steam sautéing liquid, for a lot in your Superfoods kitchen.

Suggestion: This is well worth the effort. Get in the habit of making it once a week or so. You can mix it up as needed and in response to seasonality. The important part is the regularity, proportionality and diversity inclusive of the parsley, cilantro, seaweed and mushrooms.

SUPERJUICE REJUVELAC

pure water

1/3 cup of one of the following (quinoa preferred but good to mix it up)

quinoa

kamut

buckwheat

rye

soft winter wheat berries

Steps: Soak quinoa in pure water in jar with cheese cloth and rubber band covering top for 2 hours then drain the liquid and lay jar on side. Quinoa will sprout overnight. Grind sprouted quinoa in blender with a bit of pure water and then pour into a 1 gallon glass jar and fill with pure water. Cover the jar with a towel and let stand at 65-75 degrees Fahrenheit (stable room temperature). Stir the mix once or twice a day and you can compost the floating ground grains at the top when you first stir. It is ready when it is slightly fermented and tastes a bit lemony and refreshing. Fermenting is dependent on time and temperature, it is ready when it is tart and lemony—this may be as little as 1-2 days when it is warmer, and a bit longer when it is cooler. Once ready, you can keep it in your refrigerator for about 4-5 days. This is a mildly fermented rejuvenating beverage with lots of beneficial bacteria, enzymes, bioavailable nutrients, and all sorts of other healthful

goodies. It helps to rebuild healthful bowel flora and facilitates healthful digestion and the elimination of toxins. At the early stages of fermentation, alcohol
content is negligible (very little sugar to start with in the process—we sprouted
our seeds), however, if you let it continue to ferment, with added honey or other
sugars, alcohol content will rise and it will become like bubbly champagne. This
is the living base for some of our Superfoods soups and smoothies. It is also great
plain. Drink 1-2 cups a day.

LEAFY GREEN

LIVING GREENS POWER SOUP

1 ½ cups Superjuice Rejuvelac

2 cups sprouts (any type you choose)

4 stalks celery

2 cucumbers

1 clove garlic

1 thumb sized piece of ginger

1 tsp. lemon juice

¼ tsp. sea salt

¼ cup soaked dulse

¼ small cayenne

2 avocados

2 cups greens, your choice, but lacinato kale or mustard greens are quite good

Optional: ½ cup basil

Steps: Add all ingredients, except avocado, to blender and blend on high
speed for 2-3 minutes. Add the avocado at the end—it will give a creamy texture.

Suggestion: This is a perfect lunch. You can pack it in a ball jar. Try it with
some sprouted flax crackers. You can really mix this up and get creative. You can
switch up the greens and herbs and keep it diverse. I love it with basil, but I also
like it with: lamb's quarters (aforementioned *Chenopodium album),* watercress,
purslane, dandelion greens, or any other edible green or herb. Enjoy!

SAUERKRAUT (IT'S EASY!)

5 lbs. cabbage (half green, half red)

3 tbsp. sea salt

Note: You will need a ceramic fermentation crock for this. Or you can use another vessel with at least a 1-gallon capacity, a plate that fits inside of the vessel, and a jar of water to set on top of plate to weigh it down.

Steps: Chop the cabbage finely, place in large bowl and use your hands to knead with sea salt. Let stand for 1-2 hrs. and then knead again. Pack into fermentation crock or vessel and tamp down with your hand. Then place the crock stones or plate and jar of water on the kraut to weigh it down. Basically, you want the kraut submerged in its own liquid or brine (the stones or plate and jar weigh it down pushing it under its brine). The volume of your kraut will go down slightly as it ferments, and that is fine, you want to check on it every few days to make sure it is submerged. Water content of cabbage varies and if it is dry, you might not get the water level above the stones or plate on day 1. Continue to tamp it down and if it is not submerged by day 2 (fully submerging the kraut) then add a bit of pure water with sea salt at 1 tsp. per cup. You may see mold blooms on the air-brine interface, you can skim them off, but they are normal. The kraut when submerged is protected by its brine. It will begin to get tangy at about day 3, for the recognizable kraut flavor enjoyed by many, it usually takes about two weeks. Once ready, you can pack it in jars and put them in refrigerator or cool basement. It keeps for weeks to months depending on the temperature. When it is past its prime it gets soft and tastes less pleasant.

Suggestion: I enjoy kraut over its lifecycle. Both the kraut and brine are amazing digestive tonics consisting of lots of beneficial bacteria, enzymes, bio-available nutrients, and all sorts of other healthful goodies that help to rebuild healthful bowel flora, facilitate healthful digestion and the elimination of toxins. Mix it up, you can add what you want, try grated carrots, turnips, beets or burdock. You can try other fruits, vegetables and herbs too including apples, garlic, onions, seaweed, your favorite leafy greens, caraway seeds, celery seeds, or dill seeds, even juniper berries. Have fun!

SPRING GREENS SALAD

8 oz. mesculin greens

1 medium carrot

1 medium red beet

4 large radishes

2 green onions

1 ½ lemons

2 tbsp. apple cider vinegar

2 tbsp. olive oil

Sea salt and pepper to taste

Optional: Add any type of sprout and sprinkle some chia seeds on top for a complete meal. Also, fresh herbs are great on this salad. Some of my favorites include dill, basil, oregano, and thyme. Use lots of herbs, for example, add 1 cup chopped basil or ½ cup of the others listed to the above.

Steps: In a sealable jar, mix together the olive oil, juiced lemons, apple cider vinegar, and sea salt and pepper. Top the greens with grated beet, carrot, and radishes then top with sliced green onion, dress and toss—yum! This is one of my personal favorites. Oftentimes, I will just leave off the dressing and squeeze a lemon right on with some fresh herbs and maybe a pinch of sea salt. Another awesome dressing for this salad is 4 tbsp. Nama Shoyu, 2 tbsp. flax oil, pinch of sea salt—toss well.

KALE CHIPS

2 bunches kale (green kale works great)

3 lemons

Sea salt to taste (finely ground)

Optional: Try a few cloves crushed garlic, black pepper, cayenne pepper, or even ginger—any one of these, any combo, or even all of them. Be creative and add other herbs and spices that appeal to you.

Steps: Turn your oven on, but as low as you can (you need to aim to keep it under 118 degrees to keep them raw), some ovens work like this and some don't. If this doesn't work for you, go and get a dehydrator—until then you can turn the heat up a bit, but if you do they won't be a part of your daily raw. Cut your kale to desired size (or leave whole for extra large chips!), in separate bowl, mix juiced lemons with all other ingredients except sea salt, completely coat the kale in this dressing then place dressed kale on oven rack or even cookie sheet, this is when you sea salt to taste and then "bake" them for a bit. This is the art to it all. Ideally, you want to dehydrate them, not cook them. Depending on the temperature you settle on and the type and seasonality of the kale, you might need anywhere from a few minutes to several hours or even more. Serve in a brown paper lunch bag, a fun way to enjoy your snack! Our children love these. Dehydrated kale chips are among their most preferred munchies—if not THE preferred.

KALE SAUTÉ

1 bunch lacinato kale
1 bulb (yep full bulb!) of garlic
2 tbsp. olive oil or steam sauté (see following)
Sea salt and pepper to taste

Steps: Bring the olive oil to a low-medium heat sizzle, chop the garlic into small coins and cook until the smell just begins to permeate the room, add the kale and very lightly sauté, be sure to not burn the garlic or overcook your kale—you want it to be vivid green—not brownish looking!

Suggestion: Learn how to steam sauté so as to reduce or eliminate (if you must) your use of oils in cooking. Similarly, if you use oils in cooking, you can brush or drizzle them on the pan. Do not pour! As mentioned, the best oil to cook with is coconut (given its stability with heat) followed by olive and sesame (they are also fairly stable with heat), but you can just as easily replace them with pure water, wine, or Superbroth adding a few tablespoons at a time so as to not stew what you are trying to sauté. With some of the leafy greens, you might want to get in there and use your hand to crush them up a bit as you steam sauté—this enables warming without overcooking. Steam sautéing works great—you can brown onions this way—literally (but you don't want to brown anything—this is overcooking—rather the onions should be translucent). Since we are striving to not overcook anything the steam sauté technique is a great tool in our Superfoods kitchen armamentarium.

DR. TODD'S GREENS STEAM SAUTÉ

1 bunch lacinato kale

¼ bunch red kale

¼ bunch green kale

½ bunch rainbow chard

½ bunch mustard greens

¼ small purple cabbage

½ medium red beet

1 medium Spanish black radish

4 cloves garlic

1 thumb sized piece of ginger (grated)

2 tbsp. olive oil

1 ½ cup pure water

1 tsp. sea salt

1 tsp. pepper

1 cayenne pepper (minced), optimal but optional

1 tsp. sesame seeds

1 tsp. turmeric

4 tbsp. Nama Shoyu

Optional: ¼ cup almonds added at the beginning with water

Steps: Mince garlic and cayenne; chop beet, Spanish black radish, and purple cabbage finely—add all these to water, spices, and olive oil on low heat. Then, chop all greens and throw in after water hot to touch. Smash with hand to desired texture. Keep it raw.

Suggestion: This dish goes very well with sprouted wild rice or sprouted whole grain garlic bread!

GREENS AND BEANS

2-3 heads of escarole

1 ½ cups cannellini beans (sprouted of course!)

1 bulb of garlic

2 tbsp. olive oil or steam sauté

Sea salt and pepper to taste

Steps: Bring the olive oil to a medium heat sizzle, add beans, and cook until lightly seared. Chop the garlic into small coins and cook with the beans until the smell permeates the room, add the escarole and cook until lightly wilted and slightly darker in color—don't overcook.

CABBAGE STIR FRY

1 medium to large head cabbage

2 tbsp. sesame oil or steam sauté

¼ cup almonds

2 cups brown rice

3 cups water

¼ cup Nama Shoyu

½ tsp. turmeric

1 thumb sized piece of ginger minced

Black pepper to taste (use good amount about 1 tsp.)

Optional: Shiitake mushrooms are great in this dish—you add them in prior to the almonds (add the almonds once the mushrooms are soft). Cayenne pepper and garlic are amazing spicy additions to this dish as well, you add these to the Nama Shoyu. Also, seaweed salad is a great complement. For this, soak 1 cup dried wakame in water for a few hrs. Squeeze the water out (this seaweed water is great for steam sautéing too) and toss with dressing which soaked for few hrs. as well: 1 tbsp. sesame oil, 2 tsp. Nama Shoyu, 1 tsp. sesame seeds, 2 cloves garlic minced, 1 thumb sized piece of ginger minced.

Steps: Put brown rice and water in a pot and bring to a boil; cover the pot and lower heat so the contents are at a simmer for twenty minutes (add water as needed to obtain desired rice consistency). While the rice is simmering, bring sesame oil to a low-medium heat sizzle and begin to lightly toast your almonds. Chop the cabbage into ¼ inch wide strips and sauté to your desired color and texture—still vivid green and firm. Heap the cabbage and almonds over a bed of rice. Drizzle with Nama Shoyu and serve, if you are going to add the optional cayenne and garlic, add them to the Nama Shoyu (they can be thinly sliced fresh or powdered dried, let them marinade for an hour or so).

ASIAN SALAD

1 small head purple cabbage

1 small head green cabbage

2 carrots

1 head of broccoli

1 red bell pepper

2 green onions

2 tbsp. sesame oil

½ cup unseasoned rice vinegar

¼ cup Nama Shoyu

1 tbsp. sesame seeds

Black pepper to taste (use good amount about 1 tsp.)

Optional: Grate a thumb size bit of ginger and add to dressing.

Steps: In a sealable jar, mix together the sesame oil, rice vinegar, and Nama Shoyu to be used as the dressing. Slice the cabbage into thin, slaw like strips, place in salad bowl. Grate your carrots over the cabbage. Next, cut the florets of your broccoli into small pieces, place these over the carrots. Cut the bell pepper into thin strips, again adding to the top of the salad. Top off the salad with green onion slivers. Pour the dressing over the entire salad, mix well and let marinade for one-two hours tossing at 60 minute intervals. Sprinkle with sesame seeds and serve.

ARUGULA SALAD

8 oz. arugula

1 fennel bulb

1 lemon

3 tbsp. olive oil

Sea salt and pepper to taste

Steps: Place the arugula in a salad bowl. Slice the fennel bulb as you would an onion, cutting off top and bottom, slicing in half, then placing flat sides down on the cutting board, slicing the remainder of the bulb thinly. Combine in bowl and grate one (organic!) lemon to get 1 tbsp. of zest (save the lemon, we use only the zest in this recipe). Add the zest, drizzle the olive oil, and add sea salt and pepper. Toss well and enjoy!

FORAGER'S DELIGHT

20 Fiddleheads

20 Ramps

2 tbsp. olive oil or steam sauté

1-2 lemons

Sea salt and pepper to taste

Steps: On low-medium sizzle, lightly sauté the fiddleheads (whole, not sliced) in the olive oil and a bit of water so as to steam/sauté them. Throw in the ramps (treat these as you would chives) near the end of sautéing, mix in juice of 2-3 lemons, sea salt and pepper at end, just prior to serving. Try this delicious and seasonal dish on a bed of sprouted wild rice or quinoa.

Suggestion: Steam sauté with Superbroth and white wine at a one to one ratio for an awesome twist!

FRONT YARD SALAD

6 oz. mesculin greens

2 oz. fresh dandelion greens

4 oz. fresh dill

2-3 lemons

Sea salt and pepper to taste

2 tbsp. olive oil (for an optional drizzle)

Steps: In a sealable jar, add and shake up finely chopped fresh dill, lemon juice, sea salt, and pepper to be used as the dressing. Place the mesculin greens and dandelion greens in a salad bowl, top with the dressing and enjoy.

SUPERFOODS IN A BLANKET

1-2 large heads green cabbage

1 cup cashews

½ cup pecans

½ cup walnuts

1 cup brown rice (or sprouted wild rice-you can try both!)

1 ½ cups water

½ cup quinoa

1 onion

5 medium tomatoes

Sea salt and pepper to taste

Steps: First, cook, the rice: put brown rice and 1 ½ cups of water in a pot and bring to a boil; cover the pot and lower heat so the contents are at a simmer for twenty minutes. While the rice is cooking, bring a pot of water to a boil, and dip individual cabbage leaves in the water so that the leaves are more pliable (do not overcook—just a quick dip!). Next, grind the nuts in a food processor then mix together with finely minced onion, rice and quinoa; take each cabbage leaf and plop about 1 tablespoon of the mix onto the center of the leaf and roll. Place all your rolled cabbage leaves in a baking dish and cover with sliced tomatoes and sea salt and pepper. Cover and bake at low heat until warm throughout.

KALE SALAD

2 bunches green or red kale

1 cup alfalfa sprouts

2 lemons

4 tbsp. Nama Shoyu

Sea salt and pepper to taste (you won't need much sea salt with the Nama Shoyu, but do use a good amount of black pepper)

2 tbsp. olive oil (for an optional drizzle)

Optional: A personal favorite, this salad is super on its own, or with additional toppings, such as: tomatoes, avocados, shiitake mushroom strips (marinated overnight in garlic and Nama Shoyu), olives, or sesame seeds—you name it. Olives are great, but choose wisely—sea salt brining and oil curing are traditional ways of preparing olives, stay away from canned olives (or anything in a can for that matter!).

Steps: Cut the kale into very thin strips. Add all other ingredients to kale, and mix well. Use your hands to mix making sure all the kale is well coated.

RAINBOW VEGGIES

VEGGIE GUMBO

2 cups brown rice

3 cups water

3 tbsp. sprouted chia powder

3-4 tbsp. white wine

2 tbsp. olive oil or steam sauté

1 stalk celery

1 large white onion

1 green pepper

1 red/orange/or yellow pepper

1 zucchini

3 cloves garlic

¼ tsp. cinnamon

1 tsp. dried marjoram or thyme

1 lb. okra

5-6 medium tomatoes

3 cups water (in addition to the first 3)

Sea salt and pepper to taste

Steps: First, prepare the roux: grab a small bowl and mix together the sprouted chia powder, white wine, and sea salt and pepper; put this on a low heat and warm. Set aside when done preparing. In a separate, medium heated soup pan, add the 2 tablespoons of olive oil or steam sauté the onion and celery in Super-broth, cook for approximately five minutes, then add the bell peppers, zucchini, garlic, cinnamon, marjoram, sea salt and pepper. Cook this for another five minutes, then add the final 3 cups of water, tomatoes, okra, and roux; cover and simmer on low heat for the next hour or so. While the gumbo is cooking, begin preparing the rice. Put brown rice and water in a pot and bring to a boil; cover the pot and lower heat so the contents are at a simmer for twenty minutes. The gumbo should be ladled over the hot rice; the two should be done cooking at about the same time.

Suggestion: Serve this dish with kale salad!

BUTTERNUT SQUASH SOUP

2 medium sized butternut squash
4 cups unsweetened almond milk
¼ cup grade B maple syrup
1 tbsp. cinnamon
½ cup water

Steps: Preheat your oven to 350°F; cut both the tops and bottoms off the squash, slice the squash in half vertically and scoop out the seeds; place the squash skin side up in a glass baking dish filled with the water; bake approximately twenty minutes, or until tender but firm; spoon three of the squash halves into a blender and blend with the almond milk, scoop out and cube the remaining squash half into a pot; pour blended mixture over the cubed squash, add maple syrup and bring soup to a low simmer for 10 minutes, lower heat and sprinkle on cinnamon.

Suggestion: Enjoy next to a fire on a chilly evening, or share with your family around the holiday table. Also, you can leave out all the above and just blend cubed squash with fresh squeezed orange juice to desired consistency for a RAW variation. Try with 1 tsp. of curry or 1 tsp. of cinnamon. This is a good example of easily substituting raw foods into your diet.

SPINACH MUSHROOM BARLEY RISOTTO

1 cup barley
2 cups sliced mushrooms (chanterelles, shiitake, or maitaki great here!)
8 oz. fresh spinach
4 cups Superbroth
1 white onion
1 clove garlic
3 tbsp. fresh parsley
3 tbsp. fresh chives
1 tsp. fresh oregano
1 cup white wine
3 tbsp. olive oil
Sea salt and pepper to taste

Steps: In a pan, heat half of the olive oil and sauté the onion until translucent. Add half of the Superbroth to the onions, along with the barley, oregano, sea salt, and pepper. Bring this mixture to a boil, then lower heat and simmer until most of the liquid is absorbed. For approximately the next twenty minutes, continue to add broth, ½ cup at a time, while continuously stirring. When adding the last ½ cup broth, also add the white wine, parsley, and chives. In a separate pan, add other half olive oil and sauté the mushrooms until soft. For the last five minutes of sautéing the mushrooms, add the garlic and at the last minute add the spinach. When the barley and Superbroth mixture is done cooking, put in a serving dish and top with the spinach mushroom mix.

ROCKET PASTA

1 lb. quinoa pasta
1 lb. arugula
4 large tomatoes or grape tomato equivalent (these are the best here!)
1 bulb fresh garlic
1 tbsp. olive oil or steam sauté in pure water
2 tbsp. olive oil (or Superbroth)
Sea salt and pepper to taste

Steps: Prepare the pasta as directed; while pasta is cooking, peel, cut, and sauté the garlic in 1 tbsp. olive oil (or steam sauté with Superbroth) and ½ tsp. sea salt, adding tomatoes cut to your preference near the end (tomatoes should be warmed, but retain their shape and color). Add cooked pasta to pasta bowl, mix in 2 tbsp. olive oil (or 4 tbsp. Superbroth), place arugula on pasta and pour the garlicky tomato sauce on top; mix all the contents well and enjoy, try with a nice glass of red wine and the following Nutballs.

Suggestion: Enjoy with sautéed or grilled hot banana peppers too. They are an easy and delicious way to enjoy these Superfoods superstars. Heat 1-2 tbsp. of olive oil to a low-medium sizzle and throw in some chopped garlic and a few peppers—they are ready when they are soft. Similarly, you can steam sauté peppers with a bit of Superbroth and/or white wine.

Alternatives: Quinoa pasta is versatile, for another versatile "pasta" you can use thinly sliced zucchini—it is great, try it for a raw "pasta" dish. Some awesome raw blender (throw all ingredients into blender for 1-2 minutes just prior to serving) sauces for both quinoa and zucchini pasta include:

Pesto: ½ cup (or a bit more) garlic, 1 cup pine nuts, 2 cups walnuts, 2 ½ cups basil, 2 tsp. sea salt, 2 tbsp. olive oil

Cilantro: 2 cups cilantro, 1 cup walnuts, 1 cup pine nuts, ½ cup lime juice, 2 tbsp. olive oil, small thumb sized piece of ginger

Marinara: 3 cups diced tomatoes (cherry or plum best), ¼ cup minced garlic, 1 cup basil, ½ cup red bell pepper, 2 tsp. sea salt, 2 tbsp. olive oil, ¼ cup red wine, ½ cup shallots

NUTBALLS

3 tbsp. sprouted chia powder

½ cup finely chopped onion

4 garlic cloves

1 cup cashews

½ cup pecans

½ cup walnuts

2 cups parsley

1 tsp. sea salt

1 tsp. pepper

1 tsp. red pepper flakes

Steps: Grind the nuts in a food processor, and then mix together all ingredients to make your dough. Roll the dough into little balls and steam sauté or warm in the oven on low heat just prior to serving with the above or brown/wild rice and a huge salad. Mushrooms are good with this dish too, lightly sautéed or steam sautéed maitake or shiitaki are two of our favorites.

MEXARONI

1 lb. quinoa macaroni noodles

2 cups black beans

4 oz. olives without pits

4 medium sized tomatoes

1 green bell pepper

4 cloves garlic

2 tbsp. chili powder

½ tsp. chipotle powder

3 ears corn

1 bunch cilantro

Sea salt and pepper to taste

Optional: Jalapeno peppers or even habanero peppers—thinly slice these and sprinkle them right on top to dial up the heat. These are also great soaked overnight in a bit of apple cider vinegar with a pinch of sea salt.

Steps: Cook pasta as directed. While cooking the pasta, dice the olives, mince the garlic, cube the tomatoes, cut the corn from the cobs, slice the bell pepper into strips, and finely chop the cilantro. Mix all these ingredients in with the cooked pasta when it is ready; for a muy caliente version, throw some of the hot peppers into the mix. Delicioso!

LILY'S SOUPER SOUP

2 tbsp. olive oil or steam sauté with pure water

12 medium sized tomatoes

2 large chopped onions

2 bulbs minced garlic

8 celery stalks

1 bunch chard

1 bunch kale

2 medium zucchini

1 medium yellow squash

3 carrots

1 bunch parsley

2 lemons

1 cup basil

½ cup parsley

24 cups water (ok to add 8 cups more if needed)

Dash of red wine

Sea salt and pepper to taste

Optional: Lots of fresh or dried herbs, some excellent additions include thyme and marjoram. Also, organic potatoes are great in here.

Steps: Start the base of your broth by adding the olive oil to a soup pot and sauté the onions, garlic, diced carrots, and chopped celery stalks; as the oil is absorbed and the veggies are warmed, add just a touch of red wine and a pinch of sea salt. Let this sauté on low-medium heat for three more minutes once the wine and sea salt have been added. Next add the chard, zucchini, yellow squash, and one quart of water; heat these contents to a simmer. Add all your diced tomatoes at this point, along with the remaining four quarts of water. Turn to high and bring to an almost boil, then lower to a medium heat and allow to simmer for ten minutes. Cut the lemons into quarters and finely chop the parsley and basil, add these to the soup, along with the rest of your sea salt and pepper, and simmer for an additional 20 minutes.

Suggestion: Feel free to add lentils, beans or peas. Remember to soak and sprout them though—throw them in right after the tomatoes. This soup is even better the next day, it's a good thing too since there will be lots of leftovers. This soup is a good crowd-pleaser. It is also one of our family favorites. Do get creative, you can really mix it up seasonally and it is a good warming energy food for the times of transition and cold months of winter. Serve it up with some sprouted whole grain garlic bread (drizzle of olive oil, minced garlic and parsley, sea salt and pepper). Next day preparation is easy—just add a little more water if needed along with a few handfuls of fresh greens as you warm up the soup! When working with warming soups, it becomes artful to create them as nutritive and warming as possible, therefore overcooking must be avoided, slow and steady low heat is best—also, put the soft stuff in at the end or just prior to eating. Alternatively, you can scoop a ladleful over your undressed salad or a bowl of spinach or other greens.

SUPER SANDWICH

Sprouted whole grain bread
Tomatoes
Red or Green Leaf Lettuce
Baked Beans (see following)
White Onion
Sea salt and pepper to taste

Steps: To make two sandwiches, lightly toast two slices of bread; smear some baked beans (see following) on both slices, then add a pinch of sea salt and a dash of pepper to both slices. Finally, add 2-4 slices of tomatoes, a few pieces of lettuce, some sliced onion, and serve open-faced.

BAKED BEANS

2 cups great northern beans (sprouted of course)

1 large white onion

1 cup Barbecue Sauce (see following)

Sea salt and pepper to taste

Steps:

Mix and enjoy! Warm if you want—to do so use low heat in saucepan, you can smash the beans up a bit if you prefer.

BARBECUE SAUCE (ABOUT 2 CUPS)

1 cup finely diced tomatoes

¼ cup mustard seeds (soaked in apple cider vinegar overnight)

4 cloves garlic

8 basil leaves

¾ cup chopped white onion

2 tsp. sea salt

1 tsp. black pepper

½ tsp. dried cayenne pepper or 1 small cayenne pepper

2 tsp. grade B maple syrup

2 tbsp. blackstrap molasses

Steps:

Blend at high speed!

SUMMER HARVEST SANDWICH

Sprouted whole grain bread

Garden ripe tomatoes (preferably grown by you!)

Red or Green Leaf Lettuce

1-2 tbsp. olive oil

Sea salt and pepper to taste

Optional: Thinly sliced jalapenos or habanero peppers, avocados great on here too, you can always give a drizzle of apple cider vinegar in addition to or instead of olive oil.

Steps: To make two sandwiches, lightly toast two slices of bread; lay the tomatoes on and drizzle with olive oil, sea salt and pepper to taste and then add some lettuce—serve open-faced and enjoy.

THAI GREEN CURRY

1 lb. extra firm, organic, non-GMO water packed tofu

2 cups brown rice

3 cups water

3 tbsp. coconut oil

2 cups raw coconut shreds (unsweetened and unsulfured)

2 (more) cups water

1 thumb sized piece of ginger

1 bulb minced garlic

1 large chopped onion

1 green bell pepper

1 red bell pepper

1 small eggplant

8 oz. green beans

2 tbsp. Nama Shoyu

6 tbsp. Thai curry powder—green preferred here, but could also be red or yellow (Mountain Rose Herbs has some good curry blends)

1 ½ cup basil—lots of basil!

Optional: Thai chilies for a little heat!

Steps: First, you are going to prepare your own coconut milk: add the coconut shreds and two cups of water to a blender; blend well and strain the liquid into a separate container for later use (save the coconut shreds, too). Then begin to prepare the tofu: cut the block of tofu into two long halves, stand each half upright (will resemble columns), and cut each half (column) into two triangular halves, slice the four triangular chunks of tofu into about ¼ inch slices. In a low-medium heated wok, add half of the coconut oil and 2 tsp. Nama Shoyu (the oil and Nama Shoyu should NOT splatter, if it does, lower the heat), and finally the tofu. Cook the tofu for about seven minutes on each side (it should not appear "soggy", but more crisp like, it should also not appear burned). Put brown rice and water in a pot and bring to a boil; cover the pot and lower heat so the contents are at a simmer for twenty minutes. Remove tofu from wok, add other half of coconut oil and ALL other ingredients as follows: garlic and eggplant, a minute or so later add the green beans, and additional veggies then add the curry powder, basil, and finally 2 cups coconut milk. Low-medium heat until eggplant and beans done perfectly—not overdone! Trick is to put the soft stuff in last so that they cook the shortest.

Suggestion: This is also very good with almonds or cashews in place of tofu (or leave both out). Curries are very versatile, try throwing in some bitter greens here and there as well.

BLACK BEAN AND AVOCADO SALAD

2 cups black beans

2 avocados

1 medium tomato

1 small red onion

1 bunch cilantro

2 cloves garlic

1 lemon

1 tbsp. apple cider vinegar

Sea salt and pepper to taste

Optional: Thinly sliced jalapenos or habanero peppers to add some HEAT.

Steps: In a bowl, add the beans, avocados, and tomatoes. Finely mince the garlic, onion and cilantro, add this to the bowl. On top of the salad, add the lemon juice, apple cider vinegar, and sea salt and pepper; toss the salad gently so as not to smash the avocados.

Suggestion: To eat as a burrito rather than a salad you can roll it up in collard green leaves, or sprouted grain tortillas (we like Ezekial Sprouted Grain Tortillas—they are very versatile, we even use them to make little pizzas).

KAIA'S SPECIAL CURRY

2 cups brown rice

3 cups pure water

1 ½ cups (more) pure water

1 lb. extra firm, organic, non-GMO, water packed tofu

2 tbsp. coconut oil

1 tbsp. sesame oil

1 onion

1 bulb garlic

½ small head red cabbage

1 carrot

3 stalks celery

1 red bell pepper

1 yellow bell pepper

1 bunch broccoli

1 bunch lacinato kale

½ cup Nama Shoyu

5 tbsp. curry powder (Mountain Rose Herbs has some good curry blends)

1 tsp. turmeric

Steps: First begin to prepare the tofu: cut the block of tofu into two long halves, stand each half upright (will resemble columns), and cut each half (column) into two triangular halves, slice the four triangular chunks of tofu into about ¼ inch slices. In a medium heated wok, add 2 tbsp. coconut oil and half of the Nama Shoyu (the oil and sauce should NOT splatter, if it does, lower the heat), and finally the tofu. Cook the tofu for about seven minutes on each side (it should not appear "soggy", but crisp like, it should also not appear burned). Cover the wok and keep on a low heat as you cook the rice. Put brown rice and water in a pot and bring to a boil; cover the pot and lower heat so the contents are at a simmer for twenty minutes. While the rice is cooking, prepare the vegetables by slicing into the size and cuts you desire (keeping in mind their length of cooking time). Turn the wok back to a low-medium heat, and add all of the cut veggies (hardest first), stir-fry these for a few short minutes, or until colors become more vivid (vegetables should remain firm, do not overcook them)—add the kale at the very end. Finally, add the remaining Nama Shoyu, sesame oil, curry powder, turmeric, and water, stir-fry this for about 1-2 minutes, and serve over a bed of brown rice.

RAW RAINBOW SLAW

1 red bell pepper

1 orange bell pepper

1 carrot

1 yellow squash

4 oz. green kale (minced)

1 zucchini

1 medium purple onion

4 cups shredded purple cabbage

1 thumb sized piece of ginger

2 garlic cloves

2 tbsp. sesame oil

2 tbsp. unseasoned rice vinegar

2 lemons or 1 orange (both work great here)

2 tbsp. Nama Shoyu

Sea salt and pepper to taste (be liberal with black pepper on this dish)

Steps: Add shredded cabbage to a large salad bowl. With a grater or food processor, shred the other veggies. Add this mix to the cabbage and toss. In a small sealable container, the dressing will be mixed with the remaining ingredients. Finely grate the garlic and ginger, add this to the container with the sesame oil, rice vinegar, and lemon juice. Pour the dressing over the shredded vegetables and mix well; let the slaw marinate for about 1 hour before serving.

PASTA FAGIOLI

1 lb. quinoa shells

2 cups cannellini beans

3 celery stalks

2 carrots

1 medium onion

6 cloves garlic

6-8 medium sized tomatoes

Lots of fresh herbs: bunch of basil, oregano, and parsley

or

2-4 tsp. dried basil

1-2 tsp. dried oregano

2-4 tsp. dried parsley

2 tbsp. olive oil

Sea salt and pepper to taste

Steps: Cook quinoa pasta as directed. While pasta is cooking, you will prepare the base of the soup. Begin to warm two saucepans on a medium heat. In saucepan one, add half the olive oil (or steam sauté with Superbroth) and begin to sauté the onion, carrots, and celery. When these are warmed, add the garlic and cook for approximately three minutes, then add the tomatoes (chopped), basil, oregano, and parsley and begin to simmer for the next 15 minutes. In saucepan two (which should be good and warmed up at this point), add the remaining olive oil, sea salt, pepper, and warm the cannellini beans. Be sure not to make the beans crunchy! When the beans are just right to your liking, add to saucepan one. To serve, place about ¼ cup of the pasta in individual bowls and ladle the soup over it.

ANTS ON A LOG

Celery

Raw almond butter

Raisins

Steps: Spread and fill the concave part of the celery with almond butter and sprinkle the raisins on top. Measurements for this simple treat depend on the number of kids (little or big!) you are making the snack for—it satisfies the meanest munchies!

Suggestion: Serve with a glass of iced Matcha (see Green Tea recipe section) for a light and energizing midday snack.

BALANCED PROTEINS

WHEATBERRY WALDORF SALAD

3 cups wheatberries

3-4 stalks celery

1 granny smith apple

¼ cup green grapes

¼ cup red grapes

1 bunch green onions

¼ cup dried cranberries

½ cup walnuts

2 tbsp. olive oil

¼ cup lemon juice

2 tbsp. tahini

2 tbsp. apple cider vinegar

Sea salt and pepper to taste

Steps: In a bowl or sealable jar, mix the olive oil, apple cider vinegar, lemon juice, tahini, and sea salt and pepper to make the dressing. Then, chop the celery, apples, grapes, and green onions. Finally, mix together all ingredients and cover with the dressing.

SPROUTED HUMMUS

2 cups garbanzo beans

2 tbsp. tahini paste

1 lemon

Sea salt and pepper to taste

Optional: Olives or olive oil are great in the mix too!

Steps: Add the beans and all other ingredients to a blender and blend to your liking. If you need more liquid in the blender to get it moving, add a bit more lemon.

Suggestion: Add other herbs to the mix to create various flavored hummus, for example: garlic, parsley, dill, or oregano are excellent choices. This is a condiment in our household—it is great spread on sprouted grain bread or wraps, throw on a bit of arugula and voila. You can use it to replace mayo on your sandwiches! It is also great with pretty much any other sprouted bean as well. Another we love: substitute great northern for garbanzo and apple cider vinegar for tahini.

QUINOA TABOULI

2 cups quinoa

1 bunch parsley

3 medium sized tomatoes

2 lemons

1 small red onion

5 cloves garlic

2 tbsp. olive oil

Sea salt and pepper to taste

Steps: Finely chop the parsley, tomatoes, onion, and garlic (very fine for the garlic), and add to the quinoa. Add the oil and all the juice you can get from the two lemons. Add sea salt and pepper to your liking, and mix well. Let stand for at least one to two hours before serving.

BEAN SALAD

2 cups garbanzo beans

2 carrots

1 cucumber

1 onion

2 lemons

Sea salt and pepper to taste

Optional: A few tablespoons of apple cider vinegar are a great addition. Also, try a cup of chopped parsley.

Steps: Thinly slice the carrots and toss in with beans. Cut the cucumber into four, long vertical slices, then cut these into chunks and add to the beans and carrots. Finally, add thinly diced onion and the remaining ingredients. Serve on green or red lettuce leaves.

LENTIL SOUP

1 ½ cups lentils

2 tbsp. olive oil or steam sauté

1 red onion

2 garlic cloves

1 carrot

2 celery stalks

5-6 medium to large tomatoes

8 cups water

1 bunch parsley

1 zucchini

¼ cup walnuts

Sea salt and pepper to taste

Steps: Sauté the onion, garlic, carrot, celery, and a pinch of sea salt and pepper in the olive oil, or steam sauté in Superbroth, for about 5-7 minutes. Next, add the water and chopped tomatoes and bring to a boil. At the boiling point, turn down to a simmer and add the zucchini and parsley (save a handful of chopped parsley for later). Add more water if you need, otherwise, let this simmer on low heat for the next hour. Just prior to the soup being done cooking, you will toast some walnuts by warming a pan on a medium heat and adding the walnuts until they begin to brown and become fragrant. When the soup is served, use these walnuts and a pinch of parsley as a garnish.

TROPICAL BEANS AND RICE

1 cup brown rice

1 ½ cups water

2 cups raw coconut shreds (unsweetened and unsulfured)

2 (more) cups water

1 cup black beans

2 tbsp. coconut oil

2 red onions

3-4 medium sized tomatoes

Sea salt and pepper to taste

1 fresh hot pepper of choice (habanero good, bhut perhaps too hot, but interesting!)

Steps: First, you are going to prepare your own coconut milk: add the coconut shreds and two cups of water to a blender; blend well and strain the liquid into a separate container for later use (save the coconut shreds, too). Put brown rice and water in a pot and bring to a boil; cover the pot and lower heat so the contents are at a simmer for twenty minutes. While the rice is cooking, sauté the onions and a pinch of sea salt in the coconut oil. Add the beans, tomatoes, more sea salt, and coconut milk at this point (you can add the shreds too, adding as much or as little as you'd like, depending on your texture preference); allow this to simmer until the consistency is somewhere between a soup and a stew. Be sure to have plenty of liquid with each serving; serve on a bed of rice, topped with slices of a fresh hot pepper.

BUCKWHEAT BREAKFAST

2 cups buckwheat (oat groats, or steel-cut oats good here too)

2 tbsp. grade B maple syrup

1-2 tsp. cinnamon

1-2 cups nut milk of choice—hemp or almond preferred

Optional: Throw in a handful of berries. Blueberries awesome here! You can also sprinkle some chia seeds.

Steps: Come meal time, eat the buckwheat cold or warm; to warm, put in a pot with about a quarter cup of Hemp milk and cook on a low heat for a minute or two. When serving, top with maple syrup and cinnamon plus optional berries and chia as you may prefer.

Suggestion: You can also mix the sprouted buckwheat with maple syrup, cinnamon and a handful of blueberries, raisins, goji berries or other fruit and then dehydrate for an amazing granola!

Nut Milks: You can easily make your own nut milks from your soaked and sprouted nuts—whichever you like. Just blend with 2 cups pure water, 1 cup of nuts for 1-2 minutes. You can strain or drink unfiltered. If you purchase them from store make sure they are unsweetened.

CITRUS CRANBERRY QUINOA SALAD

2 cups quinoa

¼ cup cranberries (dried or fresh)

1 orange

2 tbsp. walnut oil

¼ cup walnuts

2-3 tbsp. fresh chopped chives

Sea salt and pepper to taste

Steps: Squeeze the juice from the orange and add to the quinoa, along with the walnut oil. Finally, add the cranberries, walnuts, and chives; mix together and enjoy.

MEDITERRANEAN QUINOA SALAD

2 cups quinoa

¼ cup olives

1 medium to large tomato

½ small cucumber

½ small to medium red onion

3 cloves fresh garlic

1 tbsp. fresh chopped oregano

2 tbsp. olive oil

Sea salt and pepper to taste

Steps: Add all the ingredients; be sure the garlic is either crushed, grated, or very finely chopped, as fresh garlic can be hot—it is very good for you this way.

MEXICAN QUINOA SALAD

1 ½ cups quinoa

8 oz. black beans

2 ears corn

1 red onion

2 tomatoes

1 bunch cilantro

1 lime juiced

Sea salt and pepper to taste

Optional: 1 jalapeno pepper

Steps: Mince onion, chop tomato and cilantro and shave the kernels from the corncob, be sure to only cut the kernels and not the tough cob itself, mix all ingredients together and enjoy!

BEANS AND RICE WITH A TWIST

2 cups lentils

½ cup brown or sprouted wild rice

¾ cups water

1 bunch spinach

1 bunch scallions

2 tbsp. sesame oil

Sea salt and pepper to taste

Steps: Put the brown rice and water in a pot and bring to a boil; cover the pot and lower heat so the contents are at a simmer for twenty minutes (skip this step if using sprouted wild rice). When the rice is done cooking, warm the oil (or equivalent in Superbroth for steam sauté), sea salt, and pepper on a low-medium heated pan. Add the scallions, cook for one minute, then the lentils and rice, cooking for 3-5 minutes; try to lightly warm the rice and beans, but do not burn. Finally, add the spinach and cook until lightly wilted but vivid green.

BBQ TEMPEH

½ lb. tempeh

½ cup water

1 cup barbecue sauce (see above)

Steps: Steam the tempeh in the water to bulk it up and make it easier to crumble. When the water is evaporated, crumble the tempeh with a fork and lightly steam sauté in pure water. Finally, add the barbecue sauce and mix well.

Serving Suggestion: Serve with lettuce, tomato, and red onion on sprouted grain bread.

GRILLED ROSEMARY EGGPLANT

2-3 eggplants

½-1 dozen fresh rosemary sprigs

Sea salt and pepper to taste

1-2 tbsp. olive oil

Steps: Cut each eggplant into long halves or fourths, depending on your preference, put long slits down the center of each eggplant's pith. Leaving the skin on, brush each eggplant with olive oil; stuff rosemary sprigs in the eggplant and cover with sea salt and pepper. Place on grill and cook until skin is crispy and pith is soft and tender.

TEMPEH STRIP WRAP

½ lb. tempeh

½ cup water

Sprouted Grain Tortillas

6 tbsp. Umeboshi Plum Paste

Steps: Slice tempeh into strips; over a medium heat, steam the tempeh until water evaporates, adding more at 2 tbsp. aliquots to lightly steam sauté.

Suggestion: Spread the plum paste on tortilla, add tempeh strips and enjoy! Add toppings of your choice to the wrap: lettuce, tomato, onion, shaved carrot, avocado, alfalfa sprouts, or sliced peppers to name a few. Also, great with great northern/apple cider vinegar hummus spread with plum paste.

RAINBOW FRUITS

GREAT LAKES RICE DISH

2 cups wild rice (sprouted of course)

2 cups blueberries

Steps: Mix well and enjoy.

Suggestion: This is among my absolute favorites. Take it to your next dinner party!

FRUIT STEW

1 cup sliced avocado

½ cup pineapple

½ cup sliced plantain

½ cup sliced apple

½ cup raspberries

½ cup blueberries

2 cups orange juice

½ cup lemon juice

½ cup pitted dates

1 cup frozen strawberries

Steps: Mix fruit in bowl. Blend orange juice, lemon juice, dates and frozen strawberries. Pour over fruit and enjoy.

Suggestion: This is really good with a bit of sprouted wild grain rice and a minced jalapeno pepper in the mix.

RAINBOW FRUIT KABOBS

4 cups strawberries

1 pineapple

6 kiwis

2 cups blueberries

Steps: Cut strawberries in half, the pineapple into chunks, and the kiwis into fourths. On a skewer, place first a strawberry, then a pineapple chunk, next a kiwi coin, and finally a blueberry. Repeat this until the skewer is full of fruit. Have children make these on a rainy day with Ants on a Log (see Rainbow Veggies recipe section); also a fun (and yummy!) "craft" for a children's party. Connect them to their food.

BLUEBERRY SOUP

16 cups blueberries

8 oranges

2 oz. fresh mint

Steps: Bring blueberries and juiced oranges to a low heat simmer for few minutes. Serve hot or cold, with the mint as a garnish. This is a great dessert. Another variant is 6 apples and 2 lemons juiced, 3 tbsp. honey, 2 tsp. cinnamon and 1 tsp. lemon zest in place of the oranges and mint.

Suggestion: These "soups" are refreshing on a hot day when chilled and served cold. Or, for RAW variant: you could convert this soup into a smoothie by throwing all ingredients in a blender with 1 cup of ice and blending.

SWEET TOOTH'S SWEETHEART DELIGHT

4 cups strawberries

Raw cacao nibs

Steps: Cut strawberries vertically into "hearts", sprinkle with cacao nibs.

Serving Suggestion: Enjoy with your sweetheart and a glass or two of your favorite red wine.

OMEGA-3 FATS

FLAX CRACKERS

4 cups flax seeds

4 cups water

Spices of choice (the sky is the limit here, so roll up your sleeves and figure out what you like—one of my favorites is add ¼ cup cilantro, ¼ cup basil, ¼ cup jalapeno, all finely minced along with sea salt and pepper to taste. Another great one is a good curry blend—this is great with some of the fruit dishes.)

Steps: Soak the flax seeds and spices overnight in a sealed container. The following day, lay a thin layer of the flax paste on parchment paper on a cookie sheet, and run a butter knife through it to precut your crackers; bake this at 118°F, or your oven's lowest setting, for a few hours. The end result should be a crispy, tasty cracker that can be stored and enjoyed at a later time.

CRISPY CAPRESE

Flax crackers (see recipe above)

Sliced tomato

Walnut Pate (see following)

Capers

Sea salt and pepper to taste

Steps: Prepare the flax crackers according to the Flax Crackers recipe above. Simply top the crackers, first with Walnut Pate, then tomato, a few capers, a pinch of sea sea salt, and finally a pinch of black pepper.

WALNUT PATE

1 cup Superbroth

2 cups soaked walnuts

1 cup raw, unsoaked pine nuts

1 tbsp. garlic

1 lemon juiced

½ tsp. sea salt

½ tsp. pepper

1 tbsp. Nama Shoyu

½ cup parsley

Steps: Combine in blender and blend, then add Superbroth in increments sufficient to get blender to turn over our pate. You want it to be rather firm and well pate like. Use a rubber spatula to put into a bowl. This is an awesome spread for flax crackers, sandwiches and even fruit.

CHELLO

1 cup chia seeds

2 ½ cups pure water

1 ½ cups fresh fruit juice of choice (lemon or orange are my favorite)

Steps: Place the chia seeds in the water and allow to sit for about one-half hour. During this period, stir the chia occasionally to avoid clumping. When the chia seeds begin to resemble frogs' eggs, add the fruit juice and allow soaking overnight. The end result is a fruity, gelatinous (minus the actual gelatin) concoction which resembles jello, only with far more nutritious value. Our kids love this one—I cannot keep them out of the chia!

ISLAND TAPIOCA

½ cup chia seeds

1 cup pure water

1 cup pineapple juice (juice a pineapple)

1 cup coconut shreds (or water from two green coconuts)

1 ½ cups water (additional)—not necessary if using green coconut water

Steps: Place the chia seeds in the water and allow to sit for about one-half hour. During this period, stir the chia occasionally to avoid clumping. While these chia seeds soak, you will prepare some coconut milk; blend well the coconut shreds and additional water, then strain the liquid into a separate container (keep the shreds to add to the tapioca). When the chia seeds begin to resemble frogs' eggs, add the pineapple juice and coconut milk and allow to sit for another half-hour, again, stirring occasionally to avoid clumping. Stir in some (as much or as little) of the remaining coconut shreds just prior to serving. Add more chia if it needs to thicken, or more liquid if it's too thick.

FLAXY OATS

2 cups oat groats

1 tbsp. sprouted flax meal/powder

1 tbsp. sprouted chia powder

2 tbsp. cinnamon

¼ cup raisins

¼ cup water

1-2 cups nut milk of choice (hemp or almond are good here)

Steps: This meal is best consumed warm, so when it comes time to eat, warm the sprouted groats in a pot with the water. When serving, add the flax meal, cinnamon, and raisins as a topping, then add a splash of the nut milk of your choice.

ESSENTIALS SMOOTHIE

1 cup almond milk

1 cup hemp milk

1 cup Superjuice Rejuvelac

1 banana

2 oranges juiced (more as needed)

1 tbsp. sprouted flax meal/powder

1 tbsp. sprouted chia powder

1 tsp. vanilla

2 tbsp. greens powder, or few leaves of your favorite greens

½ cup of your favorite sprouts

Steps: Put all ingredients in a blender and blend to your desired consistency (adding extra juiced oranges if needed)—drink!

TOASTED ALMONDS

8 oz. almonds

2 tbsp. Nama Shoyu

Steps: Set a skillet to a medium-low heat and add the almonds. Cook the almonds, consistently stirring or tossing them to avoid burning, until they smell good and toasty. At this point, add the Nama Shoyu, cooking and stirring for another 1-2 minutes.

Suggestion: You can dehydrate these for an awesome raw snack! Just marinate your almonds in Nama Shoyu and dehydrate.

FUNCTIONAL FOODS

SUPER SMOOTHIE

½ cup ice

4-6 oranges juiced

1 cup nut milk (unsweetened hemp, almond or hazelnut)

1 cup Superjuice Rejuvelac

1 banana (frozen if you have one))

1 tbsp. raw cacao

1 tbsp. maca

Steps: Place all ingredients in a blender and blend to your desired consistency.

TOASTY SPROUTED SEED SNACK

4 cups sunflower or pumpkin seeds

1 tsp. sea salt

½ tsp. cinnamon

1 tbsp. olive oil

Optional: Replace the cinnamon with other herbs and spices, such as: curry, garlic, ginger, Nama Shoyu, various juices, oregano, basil, or thyme, just to name a few.

Steps: Preheat oven to lowest setting and brush a cookie sheet with the oil; spread the seeds over the cookie sheet and coat with half the sea salt and cinnamon. Bake for 10-30 minutes, then sprinkle on the rest of the sea salt and cinnamon; bake for 10-30 more minutes, or until toasty. Perfect for when you are craving something sweet and sea salty.

Suggestion: Alternatively you can dehydrate!

ROASTED PUMPKIN SEEDS

4 cups pumpkin seeds

4 tsp. sea salt

3 cups water

Steps: Add sea salt to water, stir until it dissolves completely. Put the pumpkin seeds in this saline water and allow to stand at room temp for one full day. Next day—bake as above or dehydrate.

Suggestion: Alternatively you can marinade these in garlic and Nama Shoyu—maybe even some cayenne pepper for a little added zing.

COCOA-NUT MACAROONS

2 cups raw almond meal

2 cups raw coconut shreds (unsweetened and unsulfured)

½ cup maple syrup

¼ cup raw cacao powder or nibs

Steps: Mix all ingredients together in a bowl; it should be somewhat tacky to the touch, but not gooey. Add more of any of the dry ingredients if it's too gooey. Roll into small balls, place on a cookie sheet and put in oven for several hours on its lowest temperature (or dehydrate a bit). Crack the oven door so as not to dry them out too much, you will know they are done when they are firm to the touch on the outside, but moist and soft on the inside.

CHOCOLATE ALMOND TRUFFLES

1 cup almond meal

½ cup almond butter

½ cup raw cacao powder

¼ cup grade B maple syrup (or coconut nectar)

1 tsp. vanilla

Sea salt to taste

Steps: Mix all ingredients (except half of the cacao powder, you will save this for later) well until you have the truffle "dough". Roll dough into ping-pong ball sized truffles. Dust with the cacao powder by putting the remaining powder on a plate and rolling the truffles around on it.

HONEY-COCONUT ALMOND TRUFFLES

2 cups almond meal

¼ cacao nibs

½ cup honey

¼ cup raw coconut shreds (unsweetened and unsulfured)

Steps: Mix all ingredients well until you have the truffle "dough". Roll dough into ping-pong ball sized truffles. Dust with the shredded coconut by placing the shreds on a plate and rolling the truffles around on it.

GREEN TEA

GOOD MORNIN'! MATCHA

2 cups unsweetened nut milk of choice (hemp or almond best)

4 cups water

1 tbsp. raw cacao nibs or powder

1 – 1 ½ tbsp. matcha

Steps: Mix nut milk and water together in a pot, cooking on a medium heat until it starts to look frothy and hot (do not boil or even simmer). Remove from heat, add cacao and matcha, serve in your favorite morning mug. **Note:** If you are using cocoa nibs rather than powder, put them in the pot in the very beginning as they will need to absorb liquid and soften a bit before drinking.

Suggestion: Drink slowly and reverently. Enjoy alone, with someone you love or with your whole family. We drink variants of this EVERY day.

ICED SUN MATCHA

16 cups pure water

2 tbsp. matcha

½ lemon

Steps: In a large glass jar, mix all ingredients. Place in sun for approximately one hour, then chill for one hour prior to serving. This drink can be made without warming in the sun, but who couldn't use a little more solar energy? Feel free to add a bit of raw honey or coconut nectar to sweeten things up a bit.

DARK CHOCOLATE MATCHA TRUFFLES

1 cup almond meal or sprouted chia powder

¼ cup almond butter

¼ cup cacao butter

½ cup raw cacao powder

1 tsp. vanilla

1 tbsp. matcha

Steps: Mix all ingredients (except matcha) in a blender to produce your truffle "dough." Roll the dough into the size you desire and finally coat with matcha.

JUICES

GREEN SUPREME

3 granny smith apples

4 pieces kale

½ cucumber

4 stalks celery

2 cloves garlic

1 jalapeno pepper

1 grapefruit

1 thumb sized piece ginger

Optional: Few sprigs fresh parsley and/or few sprigs fresh cilantro.

SUMMA 'DIS, SUMMA 'DAT

2 granny smith apples

2 carrots

2 stalks celery

1 beet (any color)

3-4 pieces kale

Suggestion: Depending on what you juice the veggie pulp is great dehydrated. Just spread it on a tray and dehydrate.

ORANGE YOU FEELING GOOD NOW

3 oranges

3 carrots

1 yellow beet

MAKE MINE SPICY

3 medium sized tomatoes

1 carrot

3 stalks celery

2 cayenne peppers

½ cucumber

½ bunch cilantro

PUCKER UP, MY SWEET

3 granny smith apples

½ cucumber

2 lemons

1 thumb sized piece ginger

CITRUS BLAST

3 granny smith apples

½ cucumber

2 lemons

1 orange

½ lime

1 thumb sized piece ginger

DON'T FORGET YOUR MINT

3-4 medium sized tomatoes

1 cucumber

2 carrots

4 stalks celery

3-4 cloves garlic

IMMUNITY BOOSTER

2 oranges

2 carrots

½ lemon

1 clove garlic

1 thumb sized piece ginger

A few sprigs of fresh oregano

THE TACO

2 medium sized tomatoes

5 pieces kale

3 pieces mustard greens

1 bunch fresh cilantro

1 lime

THE PURPLE PEOPLE HEALER

3 granny smith apples

2 small to medium sized red beets

2 stalks celery

½ cucumber

FLUSH IT OUT

2 cucumbers
4-5 asparagus
1 red bell pepper
1 lemon
1 clove garlic
1 bunch fresh parsley

SMOOTHIES

GREEN POWER

1 ½ cups Superjuice Rejuvelac, green coconut water, fresh squeezed orange juice, or pure water
2 tbsp. green powder
½ cup blueberries
½ banana
½ cup almonds or hempseeds plus two juiced oranges
or
1 ½ cups nut milk of choice (unsweetened hemp or almond best)
Optional: 1-2 tbsp. coconut oil or 1-2 tbsp. flax oil

VERY BERRY MACA MAGIC

1 ½ cups nut milk of choice (unsweetened hemp or almond best)
1 ½ cups Superjuice Rejuvelac, green coconut water, fresh squeezed orange juice, or pure water
1 tbsp. maca
4-5 strawberries
1 cup total of: raspberries, blackberries, and blueberries

GREEN TROPIC-COLADA

1 ½ cups nut milk of choice (unsweetened hemp or almond best)
1 ½ cups Superjuice Rejuvelac, green coconut water, fresh squeezed orange juice, or pure water
1 banana

1 kiwi

1 cup pineapple

1 tbsp. raw coconut shreds (unsweetened and unsulfured)

1-2 tbsp. coconut oil

2 tbsp. green powder

COOL PEACH PIE

1 ½ cups nut milk of choice (unsweetened hemp or almond best)

1 ½ cups Superjuice Rejuvelac, green coconut water, fresh squeezed orange juice, or pure water

1 cup peaches

½ banana

1 tsp. cinnamon

BAN-ILLA

1 ½ cups nut milk of choice (unsweetened hemp or almond best)

1 cup coconut water or pure water

2 juiced oranges

1 tbsp. maca

2 bananas

Optional: 1 ½ tsp. pure vanilla

ALMOND ADVENTURE

1 ½ cups nut milk of choice (unsweetened hemp or almond best)

1 ½ cups pure water

2 tbsp. almond butter

2 bananas

3-4 strawberries

SOAKING AND SPROUTING CHART

	Soaking Time (hours)	Sprouting Time (days)
Alfalfa	8-12	3-6
Almonds	8	n/a
Amaranth	rinse & drain	2-4
Barley	6	2
Black Beans	8-12	2
Buckwheat	6	2
Chia Seeds	1/2	
Flax Seeds	1/2	
Garbanzo Beans	8	2-3
Kamut	7	2-3
Lentils	7	3
Millet	6-10	1-5
Mung Beans	8-12	2-5
Oat Groats	6	2
Quinoa	2	1
Radish	6-12	3-6
Rye	8	3
Soybeans	2-12	2-6
Sunflower	1-4	1-5
Walnuts	4	n/a
Wheat	6-12	2-3
Wheat Berries	7	2-3
Wild Rice	9	3-5
Other Nuts	try 6	

SUPERFOODS RESOURCES
Superfoods and Supplements

Dr. Todd's Superfoods
Superfoods and Greens Powder
http://www.eatyourselfsuper.com

Earth Healers
Maca, Matcha, Cat's Claw
http://www.earthhealers.com

Awesome Foods
Raw, Packaged Superfoods
http://awesomefoods.com/

Laughing Giraffe
Raw, Packaged Superfoods
http://thelaughinggiraffe.com/

Navitas Naturals
Raw, Packaged Superfoods
http://www.navitasnaturals.com/

Hail Merry
Blond Macaroons—yum!
http://www.hailmerry.com/

Sunfood
Raw, Packaged Superfoods (great olives)
http://www.sunfood.com/

Gnosis
Raw Chocolate
http://www.gnosischocolate.com/

Go Raw
Raw, Packaged Superfoods
http://www.goraw.com/

Organic Food Bar
Active Greens
http://www.organicfoodbar.com/

Doctor in the Kitchen
Flackers, Flax Crackers
http://www.drinthekitchen.com/

Brad's Raw Chips
Kale Chips
http://www.bradsrawchips.com/

Good 'n' Raw
Raw Packaged Foods and Kale Chips
http://www.goodnraw.com/

Two Moms in the Raw
Raw Granola
http://www.twomomsintheraw.com/

Maine Coast Sea Vegetables (wakame, kelp, dulse, nori and others)
https://www.seaveg.com/shop/
Health Matters America, Organic Traditions
Raw, Packaged Superfoods—Sprouted Seed Powders
http://www.healthmattersamerica.com/

Green Foods
Green Magma
https://www.greenfoods.com/

Nature's Sunshine
Dietary Supplements and Liquid Chlorophyll
http://www.greatestherbsonearth.com/

Garden of Life
Raw, Whole Food Multivitamins and Dietary Supplements
http://www.thevitamincode.com/

New Chapter
Whole food Multivitamins and Dietary Supplements
http://www.newchapter.com/

Jade Chlorella
Chlorella
http://www.jadechlorella.com/

Amazing Grass
Wheat Grass and Superfoods Powders
http://amazinggrass.com/

SUPERFOODS MUSHROOMS

Fungi Perfecti
Medicinal and Gourmet Mushrooms and Mushroom Products
http://www.fungi.com/

WHOLE GRAIN BREAD PRODUCTS

Food for Life
Ezekiel 4:9 Sprouted Grain Breads and Wraps
http://www.foodforlife.com/

Alvarado Street Bakery
Sprouted Grain Breads and Tortillas
http://www.alvaradostreetbakery.com/

SUPERFOODS BEVERAGES

Guayaki
Yerba Mate Beverage
http://www.guayaki.com/

Sambazon
Great Acai Beverage
http://www.sambazon.com/

Steaz
Green Tea Beverage
http://steaz.com/

Mamma Chia
Chia Beverage
http://www.mammachia.com/

GT's
Kombucha
http://www.synergydrinks.com/

Pacific Foods of Oregon
Nut and Grain Beverages
http://www.pacificfoods.com/

SUPERFOODS OILS/VINEGARS, HERBS/SPICES, AND SWEETENERS

Coconut Secrets
Coconut Aminos, Coconut Nectar, Coconut Vinegar
http://www.coconutsecret.com/

Nutiva
Hemp, Coconut Oil, and Chia
http://nutiva.com/

Maple Valley Syrup
Grade B Maple Syrup
http://www.maplevalleysyrup.coop/ http://www.mastercleanser.com/

Hemp Foods
http://www.manitobaharvest.com/

Bariani Olive Oil (great olive oil!)
http://www.barianioliveoil.com/

Barlean's
Flax Oil
http://www.barleans.com/

Celtic Sea Salt
Light Grey Celtic
http://www.selinanaturally.com/

Real Salt
http://www.realsalt.com/

Bragg
Apple Cider Vinegar
http://bragg.com/
Mountain Rose Herbs
Bulk Organic Herbs, Spices and Essential Oils
http://www.mountainroseherbs.com/

HEALTH AND BEAUTY

Dr. Bronner's Magic All-One
Liquid and Bar Soaps
http://www.drbronner.com/

Nutiva
Coconut Oil
http://nutiva.com/

Living Libations
Personal Care, Essential Oils and Superfoods
http://www.livinglibations.com/

Burt's Bees
Personal and Lip Care
http://www.burtsbees.com/

Young Living
Essential Oils and Diffusers
http://www.youngliving.com/

HOUSEHOLD CLEANING SUPPLIES

Bon Ami
Nontoxic Cleaning Products
http://www.bonami.com/

Seventh Generation
Nontoxic Household Cleaning and Personal Care Products
http://www.seventhgeneration.com/

DR. TODD'S PRACTICE AND ADDITIONAL REFERENCES

Dr. Todd's Preventive, Integrative, Holistic Health Practice
http://www.drtoddpesek.com/

Dr. Todd's Healing Space Blog
http://www.healingspaceblog.com/

National Green Pages
http://www.greenpages.org/

Physicians Committee for Responsible Medicine
http://www.pcrm.biz/

Environmental Working Group
http://www.ewg.org/

American Botanical Council
http://www.herbalgram.org/

National Center for Complementary and Alternative Medicine
http://nccam.nih.gov/

Debra's List
Detoxify your home
http://www.debraslist.com/

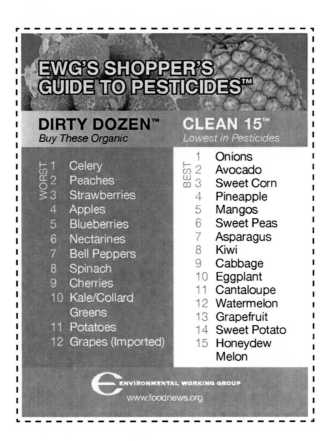

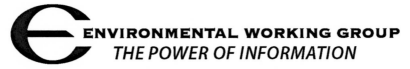

ENVIRONMENTAL WORKING GROUP
THE POWER OF INFORMATION

Headquarters 1436 U St. N.W., Suite 100 Washington, DC 20009
(202) 667-6982

Dirty Dozen and Clean Fifteen. Copyright © Environmental Working Group,
www.ewg.org. Reprinted with permission.

Why Should You Care About Pesticides?

The growing consensus among scientists is that small doses of pesticides and other chemicals can cause lasting damage to human health, especially during fetal development and early childhood. Scientists now know enough about the long-term consequences of ingesting these powerful chemicals to advise that we minimize our consumption of pesticides.

What's the Difference?

EWG research has found that people who eat five fruits and vegetables a day from the Dirty Dozen™ list consume an average of 10 pesticides a day. Those who eat from the 15 least contaminated conventionally-grown fruits and vegetables ingest fewer than 2 pesticides daily. The Guide helps consumers make informed choices to lower their dietary pesticide load.

Will Washing and Peeling Help?

The data used to create these lists is based on produce tested as it is typically eaten (meaning washed, rinsed or peeled, depending on the type of produce). Rinsing reduces but does not eliminate pesticides. Peeling helps, but valuable nutrients often go down the drain with the skin. The best approach: eat a varied diet, rinse all produce and buy organic when possible.

How Was This Guide Developed?

EWG analysts have developed the Guide based on data from nearly 89,000 tests for pesticide residues in produce conducted between 2000 and 2008 and collected by the U.S. Department of Agriculture and the U.S. Food and Drug Administration. You can find a detailed description of the criteria EWG used to develop these rankings and the complete list of fruits and vegetables tested at our dedicated website, www.foodnews.org.

Learn More at FoodNews.org

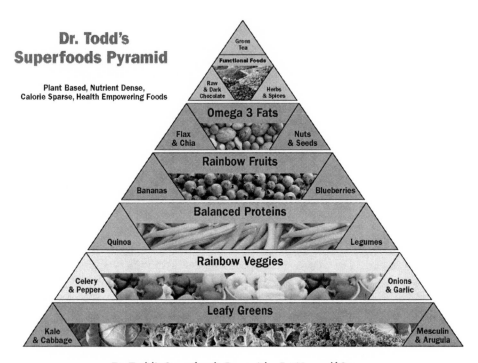

Dr. Todd's Superfoods Pyramid—Eat Yourself Super

BUY A SHARE OF THE FUTURE IN YOUR COMMUNITY

These certificates make great holiday, graduation and birthday gifts that can be personalized with the recipient's name. The cost of one S.H.A.R.E. or one square foot is $54.17. The personalized certificate is suitable for framing and will state the number of shares purchased and the amount of each share, as well as the recipient's name. The home that you participate in "building" will last for many years and will continue to grow in value.

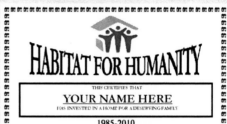

Here is a sample SHARE certificate:

THIS CERTIFIES THAT

YOUR NAME HERE

HAS INVESTED IN A HOME FOR A DESERVING FAMILY

1985-2010

TWENTY-FIVE YEARS OF BUILDING FUTURES
IN OUR COMMUNITY ONE HOME AT A TIME

1200 SQUARE FOOT HOUSE @ $65,000 = $54.17 PER SQUARE FOOT
This certificate represents a tax deductible donation. It has no cash value.

YES, I WOULD LIKE TO HELP!

I support the work that Habitat for Humanity does and I want to be part of the excitement! As a donor, I will receive periodic updates on your construction activities but, more importantly, I know my gift will help a family in our community realize the dream of homeownership. **I would like to SHARE in your efforts against substandard housing in my community!** *(Please print below)*

PLEASE SEND ME _____ SHARES at $54.17 EACH = $ $_____

In Honor Of: _____

Occasion: (Circle One)   HOLIDAY   BIRTHDAY   ANNIVERSARY

OTHER: _____

Address of Recipient: _____

Gift From: _____ *Donor Address:* _____

Donor Email: _____

I AM ENCLOSING A CHECK FOR $ $_____ PAYABLE TO HABITAT FOR HUMANITY <u>OR</u> PLEASE CHARGE MY VISA OR MASTERCARD *(CIRCLE ONE)*

Card Number _____ Expiration Date: _____

Name as it appears on Credit Card _____ Charge Amount $ _____

Signature _____

Billing Address _____

Telephone # Day _____ Eve _____

PLEASE NOTE: Your contribution is tax-deductible to the fullest extent allowed by law.
Habitat for Humanity • P.O. Box 1443 • Newport News, VA 23601 • 757-596-5553
www.HelpHabitatforHumanity.org

CPSIA information can be obtained at www.ICGtesting.com
Printed in the USA
BVOW062312010312

284246BV00001B/8/P